Occupational Therapy in Oncology and Palliative Care

Occupational Therapy in Oncology and Palliative Care

Edited by **Jill Cooper**

Head Occupational Therapist
The Royal Marsden NHS Trust

Clephane Hume: Consulting Editor in Occupational Therapy

SINGULAR PUBLISHING GROUP, INC.
SAN DIEGO, CALIFORNIA

British Library Cataloguing in Publication Data
A catalogue record for this book is available from the British Library.

ISBN 1 86156 015 X

Singular Number 1-56593-884-4

Printed and bound in the UK by Athenaeum Press Ltd,
Gateshead, Tyne & Wear

Dedicated to Peter, Joyce and Stanley.

Contents

Foreword

Recent years have seen amazing developments in health care –
particularly in oncology and palliative care. In the mid-1940s radiotherapy was still in its infancy. It produced promising results but the
public, and indeed many health professionals, viewed it with some
trepidation. Chemotherapy has only been available to cancer
patients since the 1960s. It has also been promising but patients
found it frightening until very recently, not least because of the seem-
ingly inevitable side effects which they often described as being
worse than the disease itself. Both of these treatments have been
developed and are now more acceptable to patients. New anti-
emetic drugs continue to appear, offering relative freedom from the
nausea and vomiting associated with chemotherapy. Other drugs are
able to improve appetite and slow down cancer cachexia. The use of
surgery in treating malignant disease has also changed, with the
introduction of new operating techniques, the growth of thoracic
surgery, the use of organ transplants, developments in immunother-
apy, and exciting prophylactic orthopaedic procedures for spinal
stabilization and bone metastasis. Some of the childhood malignan-
cies are now curable and, even when they cannot be cured, worth-
while long-term remissions are commonplace for people of all ages.

Developments in palliative care have been dramatic. The first
modern hospice was only opened as recently as 1967 but today, in the
United Kingdom alone, there are 217 such units or services, ever
more home care services, a growing number of day hospices, and an
incredible increase in the number of palliative care teams serving
patients with advanced cancer in general hospitals and oncology
centres – from four in the early 1970s to over 250 in 1996. There have
been many developments since the mid-1980s: the new specialities of
palliative medicine and palliative care nursing have been recognized,
many professional associations representing a spectrum of disciplines

caring for these patients have been started, and many peer-reviewed professional journals (so essential to record the ever-increasing volume of clinical research taking place in this exciting field) have been born.

Each advance has given rise to a new vocabulary, from 'tumour bulk' to 'mitotic index', from 'oncogenes' to 'host-graft reaction'. One word that has not been sufficiently used is 'rehabilitation'. To many it seems a contradiction in terms to speak in the same breath of 'rehabilitation' and a terrible life-threatening illness (and no one would deny that cancer remains that for most patients). For too long we have regarded the aim of rehabilitation as the restoration of full health and strength – as a means of returning patients to full activity and well-being so that they can be physically and socially well and economically useful again. Much of the credit for reminding us of the true meaning of rehabilitation must go to occupational therapists and physiotherapists who, working alongside doctors and nurses, have helped to develop the concepts of team caring and sharing. They are redefining the priorities of cancer and palliative care, recognizing that it is as important to maintain the quality of life as it is to save or prolong life. They are enabling more patients to live fuller lives than anyone ever thought possible and are helping many to spend long periods at home, even where the disease has become life-threatening or even terminal. Occupational therapists have revolutionized the treatment of cancer with their informed knowledge of malignant disease and its management, their highly developed appreciation of how to utilize every means available to restore quality in the face of loss, and their ability to do so not only with skill but with sensitivity and compassion.

More thought needs to be given to advanced training in occupational therapy for oncology and in palliative care. Opportunities for research are legion with countless issues waiting to be addressed. Those of us who have learned so much from colleagues in occupational therapy, and who have seen so many lives transformed, look forward to the day when every oncology service and every specialist palliative care unit has at least one occupational therapist in the team. Our patients deserve nothing less.

It has been an honour to contribute to this book and to know and work with some of its contributors. Occupational therapists, whether qualified or still in training, need to learn how their contribution to the treatment of cancer and palliative care is indispensable and how such work is exciting and rewarding. This is a publication that is long overdue.

Derek Doyle
Vice-Chairman, National Council for Hospice and
Specialist Palliative Care Services

Preface

Occupational Therapy in Oncology and Palliative Care aims to encourage and help students and clinicians in a challenging field by examining some of the broad issues confronting them. It does not provide specific solutions for specific problems. Physical dysfunctions, psychosocial difficulties and psychological coping mechanisms differ from individual to individual and occupational therapists need to use their core skills – and especially their problem-solving skills – to analyse each case as it arises. The book therefore examines these core skills and discusses their application.

Working with clients who have cancer or who are in the palliative stages of a disease involves considering their ability to survive and, if their illness is terminal, it means assessing how to help them and their carers achieve the best quality of life in the remaining time. A variety of aspects of this complex task form the focus of this book, ranging from anxiety management to symptom control and the assessment of clients and their carers for equipment such as wheelchairs or commodes.

The first chapters begin with an introduction to cancer terminology, treatments, side effects and related matters. This is followed by a discussion of the principles of assessment and treatment, first in general terms and then with specific reference to cancer patients. Subsequent chapters deal with more specialized areas of occupational therapy such as paediatric oncology and hospice day care. Finally, aspects of professional practice are discussed, such as models, note-keeping, standards and audits.

There are a number of appendices providing general information including specimen order forms, details of relaxation techniques, useful addresses, case studies and advice on the prevention of cancer. A glossary has also been provided to explain some of the more technical terms used in the book.

Occupational Therapy in Oncology and Palliative Care will assist both graduates and clinicians who are new to oncology and palliative care. It is hoped that it will help them to use their professional skills to enable their clients to achieve optimum functional independence.

Acknowledgements

I wish to thank the following for permission to use copyright material.

Harper & Row for Table 1.1: nomenclature of connective tissue and muscle tumours.

Cancer Research Campaign for Figure 1.1: number of cancer deaths for men and women in the UK, 1993.

Blackwell Scientific Publications for Table 1.2: aetiology of cancer.

SPCK Holy Trinity Church for Fig. 2.1: normal patterns of bereavement.

Disabled Living Foundation for Fig. 3.1: patient-handling sling.

Equipment for Disabled People for Fig. 3.2: grabrails.

Disabled Living Foundation for Fig. 3.3: hoist.

National Council for Hospice and Specialist Palliative Care Services for Table 4.1: Common pain problems in adult cancer patients.

Judith Waterlow for Fig. 4.1: the Waterlow Scale.

Williams and Wilkins for Fig. 10.1: human occupations model (an adaptation).

Warren Pearl Marie Curie Centre, Day Care for Fig. 10.3: Day Care timetable.

Blackwell Scientific Publications for Fig. 12.1: synthesis of Donabedian and Wilson.

Canadian Journal of Occupational Therapy for Fig. 12.2: Canadian occupational performance measure.

I would also like to thank:

Revd Tom Gordon for his advice on dealing with loss;

Dr Alison Laver-Ingram, lecturer in occupational therapy, for her advice on feeding problems;

Dr Jane Maher, consultant oncologist, Mount Vernon Centre for Cancer Treatment, for information on radiation-induced brachial plexopathy;

Dr Agnes Kocsis, clinical psychologist, for her advice on cognitive difficulties;

Warren Pearl Marie Curie Centre for the statements on philosophy of care;

National Council for Hospice and Specialist Palliative Care Service for information on standards and audit;

Blackwell Scientific Publications and The Royal Marsden NHS Trust for occupational therapy standards and audit for patients undergoing palliative care;

Occupational Therapy Department, St George's NHS Trust, for priorities of care and furniture measurement form;

Merton and Sutton NHS Trust Wheelchair Service for the pressure relief cushion assessment forms;

College of Occupational Therapists, UK, for information on core skills and professional issues.

I would like to thank the following for their contributions and helpful comments:

Patsy Aldersea, Sandra Behan, Josalyn Berkeley, Denise Brady, Ann Brdarevic, Adine Callaghan, Gillian Craig, Debbie Fenlon, Katie Hart, Camilla Hawkins, Karen Jepsen, Sasha von Lieven Knapp,

Sarah Penfold, Revd James Smith, Val Smith, Dr Maggie Watson, former and present staff, colleagues and patients at The Royal Marsden NHS Trust.

Jill Cooper

Contributors

Jill Cooper, DipCOT SROT, Head Occupational Therapist, The Royal Marsden NHS Trust, London.

Jo Bray, DipCOT SROT, Head Occupational Therapist, Warren Pearl Marie Curie Centre, Solihull, West Midlands, UK.

Shona Bruce Crosthwaite, MSc DipCOT SROT, formerly Malcolm Sargeant funded occupational therapist.

Gillian McVey MSc DipCOT SROT, Head Occupational Therapist, HIV/AIDS, Chelsea and Westminster Hospital, London.

Introduction

Jill Cooper

This book is primarily concerned with the role of occupational therapy in the treatment of cancer. Occupational therapy can, in fact, contribute to the treatment of any chronic condition or non-curable disease. It is the task of the occupational therapist to treat the client's functional problems as they arise irrespective of the origin of the illness, although the diagnosis can affect both the prognosis and the urgency with which the occupational therapy service is needed.

Occupational therapists aim to maintain their clients in their own homes by controlling symptoms and providing home-care support, including training. They can assist in any stage of an illness from the initial task of health promotion to the later stages when disabilities may be more severe. They take a holistic, flexible, client-centred approach, and this is constantly reassessed according to the needs of clients and their carers. Areas in which occupational therapists make a contribution include:

- assisting clients with activities for the treatment of physical dysfunction;
- retraining clients in personal and domestic activities that are necessary for daily living;
- the assessment of seating needs and the prescription of wheelchairs;
- retraining clients in order to help them with cognitive and perceptual dysfunction;
- splinting to prevent deformities and to control pain;

- home assessments;
- referral to social services for home assessment and provision of equipment;
- lifestyle management – investigating hobbies and leisure pursuits;
- provision of advice on and education about relaxation techniques and energy conservation;
- provision of support and education for carers; and
- assistance with psychological adjustment and goal-setting related to loss of function.

Occupational therapists also enable clients by making them aware of the services that are available, even if those services are not required immediately. If clients know what is available and where to obtain it they can make use of appropriate services at a later date if necessary. This prevents them struggling needlessly and helps them to help themselves.

As the assessment of each client covers many aspects of life it is necessary for an occupational therapist to establish a good rapport with him or her. Even the simplest of interactions can raise numerous issues. It may be that all the occupational therapist does is provide a padded bathboard to help a client wash comfortably. The ramifications of this include:

- giving the client the choice of when to bath rather than the client having to wait for an attendant;
- reducing anxiety;
- promoting self-esteem;
- dignity;
- privacy;
- avoiding being dependent on others;
- safety.

The range of services available to people suffering from cancer, or any life-threatening illness, is changing dramatically and there is now a firm emphasis on multidisciplinary teamwork rather than on the medical and nursing staff alone. Occupational therapy is one part of the service provided by the multidisciplinary team and it relies on early referral, ongoing communication and the support of all its members if it is to work efficiently and effectively. In particular, the entire team needs to be aware of the changing needs of the client as the disease progresses.

In the fields of oncology and palliative care, the multidisciplinary or interdisciplinary team is likely to comprise the following staff:

- occupational therapist
- nursing staff
- physiotherapist
- dietitian
- speech therapist
- chaplaincy
- community liaison

- surgical appliances officer
- home care nurse/Macmillan nurse
- art therapist
- social worker
- medical staff
- psychiatrist/psychological support.

Jackson and Davies (1995) make the point that:

> At the outset, role definitions must be made clear and boundaries defined. This process should give each member of the team a clear understanding of the others' roles, skills and capabilities. Ongoing staff support and training are essential to avoid the feeling of isolation.

Occupational therapists find that defining their own role clearly helps them to cope with working with the acutely or terminally ill. It should, however, be borne in mind that while clear role identification enables health care workers to achieve their goals, this should not prevent people from working together where boundaries overlap and blur.

Providers of oncological and palliative care are increasingly employing occupational therapy services as there is an increasing emphasis on supporting clients in their own homes. Occupational therapists have taken the initiative to increase networking and communication within the profession by establishing the Specialist Section of HOPE (HIV/AIDS, Oncology Palliative Care and Education). This, together with the increasing number of palliative care modules in postgraduate education, indicates a growing need for occupational therapists and the expansion of education in these areas.

Chapter 1
What is Cancer?

Jill Cooper

Cancer is a general term applied to tumours or growths. Body cells normally regenerate and die continually so the number of cells remains constant. When cells become cancerous there is an abnormal and uncontrolled increase in their growth rate, resulting in a mass, tumour or growth. The tumour may be benign or malignant.

Benign tumours grow slowly and do not recur after excision. They can still be life-threatening if untreated as they can affect vital organs. They are usually curable if they are treated early.

Malignant tumours can infiltrate and destroy the normal tissues surrounding them and spread to other sites.

Metastases occur when the primary tumour spreads by invading surrounding cells via the bloodstream or lymphatic system. These deposits are also referred to as *secondaries*.

There are some additional important terms that need to be defined at the outset to avoid possible confusion. The term *occupational therapist* refers to occupational therapy staff at all levels, whether they are state-registered occupational therapists, associates, technicians, helpers or students. The terms *oncology, anaplasia, neoplasms* and *tumours* can all be used instead of the word *cancer*.

Terminal refers to clients who are in the last few days of life. A diagnosis of cancer does not necessarily mean that the disease will become 'terminal', and the phrase *terminal illness* can refer equally well to the end stages of neurological, viral or respiratory illness.

Palliation refers to the alleviation of symptoms rather than the attempt to cure disease and it is associated with the advanced stages of all diseases, including cancer and HIV/AIDS. The World Health Organization defines 'palliative care' as 'the active total care of patients and their families by a multiprofessional team when the patient's disease is no longer responsive to curative treatment' (World

Health Organization, 1990). In occupational therapy intervention there is not a finite point between acute and palliative care. The focus may change from one to the other as the client progresses or deteriorates. Symptoms are approached in a similar manner and treatment depends on the client's functional status.

Other technical terms are given in the glossary.

Dysfunction may be the result of the tumour and/or the side effects of medical intervention such as chemotherapy or radiotherapy.

Classification of tumours

Tumours are classified according to histogenesis – the tissues and cells where they originate. Cancers are often described in terms of *degrees of differentiation*. Gowing and Fisher (1988) explain that a tumour's degree of differentiation is 'the extent to which [it] resembles the normal tissue from which it is derived'. If it closely resembles the normal tissue it is well differentiated, otherwise it is poorly differentiated. When tumour cells lose all similarity to the corresponding normal tissue they are referred to as *undifferentiated* or *anaplastic*.

Tumours of the muscle and connective tumours might be classified as in Table 1.1.

Table 1.1: Nomenclature of connective tissue and muscle tumours

Tissue of origin	Benign tumours	Malignant tumours
Fibrous tissue	Fibroma	Fibrosarcoma
Adipose (fatty) tissue	Lipoma	Liposarcoma
Bone	Osteoma	Osteosarcoma
Cartilage	Chondroma	Chondrosarcoma
Connective tissue near joints	Benign synovioma	Synovial sarcoma
Blood vessel endothelium	Haemangioma	Haemangiosarcoma
Lymph vessel endothelium	Lymphangioma	Lymphangiosarcoma
Smooth muscle	Leiomyoma	Leiomyosarcoma
Striated muscle	Rhabdomyoma	Rhabdomyosarcoma

From Tiffany (1989).

Commonest forms of cancers

Souhami and Tobias (1995) state that one in 250 men and one in 300 women are diagnosed as suffering from cancer every year. As the elderly population grows and as more people with cancer live longer due to better treatment there are increasing numbers of people with residual dysfunction and disabilities who require occupational therapy. Whilst the treatment and management of the primary tumour have obviously been the main focus of medical input, metastatic spread is still the main cause of death. This spread often develops before diagnosis and treatment have begun, so prognosis is not altered by treatment of the primary cancer.

The Cancer Research Campaign (CRC) (1995) explains that data concerning the incidence of cancer and mortality data have to be estimated for much of the world's population because of difficulties in collecting reliable information. From the information available to the Campaign, it estimates that among the newly registered cases of cancer worldwide, the 10 commonest are cancers of the lung, stomach, breast, colorectal cancers, cancer of the cervix uteri, oral cancer, lymphoma, liver cancer and cancers of the oesophagus and prostate.

The majority of newly registered cases in the developed countries are lung cancer, colorectal cancer, and cancer of the breast, stomach and prostate. In developing countries, by contrast, the majority of newly registered cases are cancer of the stomach, lung, cervix, oral cancer and breast cancer.

Figure 1.1 gives statistics on the number of deaths for males and females in the UK in 1993.

People who are treated when their cancer is at an early stage invariably have a better chance of survival.

Aetiological factors

Souhami and Tobias (1995) have listed some aetiological factors and the cancers to which they relate. These are given in Table 1.2.

Table 1.2: Aetiology of cancer

Ionizing irradiation	
Atomic bomb and nuclear accidents	Acute leukaemia and breast cancer
X-rays	Acute leukaemia, squamous cell skin carcinoma
Ultraviolet irradiation	Basal cell carcinoma, squamous cell skin carcinomas, melanoma
Backgound irradiation	Acute leukaemia
Inhaled or ingested carcinogens	
Atmospheric pollution with polycyclic hydrocarbons	Lung cancer
Cigarette smoking	Lung cancer, laryngeal cancer, bladder cancer
Asbestos	Mesothelioma, bronchial carcinoma, chromates, lung cancer
Arsenic	Lung cancer, skin cancer
Aluminium	Bladder cancer
Aromatic amines	Bladder cancer
Benzene	Erythroleukaemia
Polyvinyl chloride	Angiosarcoma of the liver

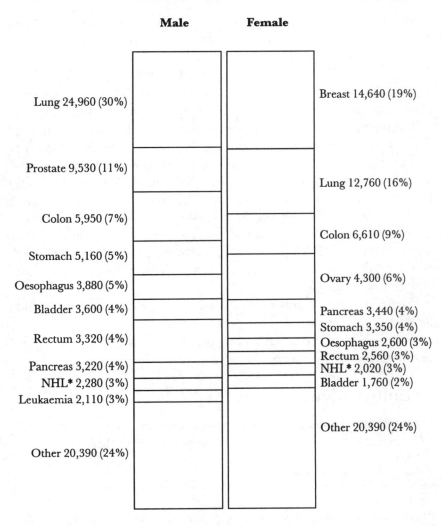

Male   **Female**

Lung 24,960 (30%)

Prostate 9,530 (11%)

Colon 5,950 (7%)

Stomach 5,160 (5%)

Oesophagus 3,880 (5%)

Bladder 3,600 (4%)

Rectum 3,320 (4%)

Pancreas 3,220 (4%)

NHL* 2,280 (3%)

Leukaemia 2,110 (3%)

Other 20,390 (24%)

Breast 14,640 (19%)

Lung 12,760 (16%)

Colon 6,610 (9%)

Ovary 4,300 (6%)

Pancreas 3,440 (4%)

Stomach 3,350 (4%)

Oesophagus 2,600 (3%)

Rectum 2,560 (3%)

NHL* 2,020 (3%)

Bladder 1,760 (2%)

Other 20,390 (24%)

All cancers 84,400 (100%)   All cancers 77,370 (100%)

*Non-Hodgkins Lymphoma.

Figure 1.1: Number of cancer deaths for men and women in the UK, 1993

The influence of diet is constantly being researched. High fat intake has been linked to high incidences of cancer. This is incon-clusive, however, since those affected tend to live in more heavily industrialized areas where there may also be high calorie and protein intake.

Watson and Ramirez (1991) state that the studies purporting to examine the role of stressful life experiences in the onset of cancer are flawed and that they cannot provide good evidence for such a relationship.

Symptoms of cancer

Initial signs of cancer include:

- a lump;
- a sore that does not heal (including one in the mouth);
- a mole that changes in shape, size or colour, or any abnormal bleeding.
- persistent problems of any kind, such as a persistent cough, persistent hoarseness, a change in bowel or urinary habits or an unexplained weight loss.

Once an individual has presented to his or her general practitioner with a lump or other symptoms that might indicate cancer, the general practitioner refers him or her to the local general hospital for a consultation.

Hanratty and Higginson (1994) list the symptoms requiring attention in the advanced stages of the illness as:

pain	weakness and tiredness
dyspnoea	poor mobility
cough	lymphoedema
nausea and vomiting	ascites
intestinal obstruction	hypercalcaemia
constipation	dehydration
diarrhoea	haemorrhage
dysphagia excessive	sweating
hiccup	pruritus
anorexia	disfigurement
cachexia	smell
pressure sores	insomnia
fungating lesions	fear and anxiety
sore and dry mouth	depression
urinary problems	confusion

Despite these symptoms, many clients progress well with treatment and continue to live productive and independent lives.

Investigations

Screening

Chamberlain (1988) concludes that the value of screening for breast and cervical cancer has been established, although in the case of breast cancer this is only certain for females of more than 50 years of age. Once females embark on the cervical screening programme they are screened as often as resources allow. Investigations continue into the efficacy of screening for other sites though trials have failed to show any benefit for lung cancer screening. Testicular cancer has such a good cure rate that screening could only enhance prognosis.

Staging

Staging identifies the stage that the disease has reached – whether it is in an early or an advanced form. Staging is one way of establishing the factors that are likely to influence prognosis in any individual patient. Souhami and Tobias (1995) have indicated that the purposes of careful staging of tumour spread are:

- to give appropriately planned treatment to the individual patient;
- to be able to give the best estimate of prognosis;
- to compare similar cases in assessing and designing trials of treatment;
- to impose discipline in the accurate documentation of the initial tumour;
- to assist our understanding of tumour biology.

The 'TNM' system is commonly used, although not in leukaemias or in lymphoma where the disease is generalized. This evaluates:

T – the size, site and depth of the primary tumor's invasion depending on type of tumour. This is evaluated on a scale ranging from T1 to T5;

N – lymph node spread, evaluated on a scale from N1 to N5;

M – the presence of distant metastases, evaluated on a scale from M1 to M5.

Tobias (1995) gives an example:

> T3, N1, M0 laryngeal cancer would imply a primary tumour suffi-
> ciently locally advanced to have fixed the vocal cord and early lymph
> node invasion causing a palpable swelling in the neck but no evidence
> of metastatic spread.

Other investigations

The client will need to undergo many of the following investigations in order for diagnosis and treatment procedures to be established.

- X-ray
- Blood count
- Enzymes
- Ultrasound. This is mainly used for the abdomen and soft tissues, particularly the liver. It is non-invasive, cheap and quick.
- Computerized tomography (CT) scan. This demonstrates the distortion or enlargement of an organ or a change in density and thus shows the extent of infiltration of primary tumours and delineates metatastic spread to adjacent lymph nodes and other structures.
- Magnetic resonance imagery (MRI). This is used particularly for spinal cord, brain and sarcoma and evidence of bone metastases.
- Isotope scanning.
- Surgery – aspiration cytology, needle biopsy and CT guided fine needle biopsy. Biopsies reveal the type of tumour, the level of differentiation and the degree of invasion.

Treatments/interventions

Surgery

Westbury (1988) classified cancer surgery as follows:

- Primarily curative. Local control of cancer is essential as the primary site either causes or contributes substantially towards death.
- Adjuvant – used alongside chemotherapy and radiotherapy.
- Palliative. For example, surgery might be used if a tumour compresses other areas or if it is necessary to block a nerve for pain control.
- Emergency – to remove life-threatening obstruction.
- Reconstructive. For example, surgery may be undertaken on skin or muscle flaps to supplement an underlying plastic prosthesis for cosmetic purposes.
- Diagnostic and staging. Biopsy provides a specimen from which a diagnosis can be made.
- Prophylactic. For example, laser destruction can remove pre-malignant lesions thus preventing further tumour growth.
- Surgery for metastases. Metastasectomy (removal of metastases) takes place alongside chemotherapy and has great palliative value.
- Surgery for vascular access. A Hickman line can be inserted to provide chemotherapy; the central intravenous line is inserted until it lies in the superior vena cava or right atrium and chemotherapy can be administered.

Laser surgery is useful in accessible head and neck cancers and colorectal liver metastases.

Radiotherapy

Radiotherapy is the use of high-energy rays to kill cancer cells. It is often able to control the tumour with minimal physiological disturbance. There are different types of radiotherapy, and these should be matched to the individual's diagnosis and needs. The factors taken into account when planning radiotherapy include:

- the type and stage of the tumour;
- the localization of the tumour;
- adjacent normal structures.

Duchesne and Horwich (1988) explain that:

> . . . the total dose of radiotherapy which can be given to eradicate a tumour is obviously limited by the tolerance of the normal tissues so that unacceptable damage is avoided.

Detailed planning is needed and this may include the preparation of an individually moulded cast. The client wears this during radiotherapy and it positions him or her correctly. The exact positioning and dosage of radiotherapy is calculated. Radiographers position the client on the couch, sometimes using marks made on the skin in indelible ink, and the radiation beam is switched on. Radiographers watch through a window or use a closed-circuit television and there is an intercom for communication with the client.

Radiotherapy may be used alone or together with surgery or chemotherapy. In addition to treating localized tumours it is often used as a palliative treatment to relieve pain or bleeding, or to suppress bone metastases which are developing into pathological fractures. Often clients find that they feel worse before the symptoms are alleviated.

Side effects can include:

- fatigue and malaise, sometimes caused by bone marrow depression;
- anorexia, nausea and vomiting;
- alopecia;
- inflammation around the site being treated. This can cause internal side effects such as mucositis, oesophagitis, laryngitis, diarrhoea, cystitis;
- anxiety and altered body image.

Chemotherapy

This is the use of cytotoxic drugs to kill cancer cells. The drugs enter the bloodstream and destroy cancer cells by interfering with the cells' ability to grow and divide. Although normal cells can be damaged, most healthy tissue grows back again.

Chemotherapy can be used in the following ways:

- as the only or most important treatment for cancer;
- to shrink tumours or to enhance the effectiveness of surgery or radiotherapy;
- it can be used after radiotherapy or surgery to eliminate remaining tumour cells and reduce risk of relapse;
- it can be used to treat a patient who has relapsed following initial successful treatment;
- it has a palliative function, relieving symptoms.

Chemotherapy may be administered orally, intravenously, intramuscularly or intracavity. The dosage and the frequency of dosage depend on the disease and the individual.

Most cytotoxic drugs are toxic to bone marrow and so can lower the blood cell count. Blood tests are, therefore, necessary to ensure the body is strong enough to cope. If very high doses of chemotherapy have to be used, bone marrow is taken from the client before treatment and returned later. In this way, marrow is not affected by the drug and, once it has been reintroduced to the patient, it assists in recovery.

Short-term side effects may include anorexia, nausea and vomiting, stomatitis, pain at the tumour site or in the jaw area, malaise, flu-like symptoms (including fever), chemical cystitis, haematuria, red/green urine, constipation and diarrhoea.

Long-term side effects may include bone marrow depression, alopecia, skin reactions, nail ridging, thrombophlebitis, pulmonary fibrosis, congestive cardiac failure, liver dysfunction, renal toxicity, neurological problems, central nervous system toxicity, sexual dysfunction and peripheral neuropathies.

Bone marrow transplantation (BMT)

The purpose of bone marrow transplantation is to eradicate deficient or malignant marrow. During the course of treatment both bone marrow and disease are eradicated by chemotherapy and/or radiotherapy, so bone marrow is restored afterwards in the following ways:

- syngenic replacement – the donor and the recipient are genetically identical;
- allogenic replacement – the donor and the recipient are from the same species;
- autologous replacement – the patient's own marrow is used following cytotoxic therapy.

BMT is used to treat:

- acute myeloid leukaemia (AML);
- acute lymphoblastic leukaemia (ALL);
- chronic myeloid leukaemia (CML);
- neuroblastoma, when not cured by initial chemotherapy;
- in severe immune deficiency states, thalassaemia major and sickle cell anaemia;
- aplastic anaemia.

Patients treated with BMT are likely to become very tired and weak and will often be in isolation while the body is immunosuppressed.

Action points

1. Using the recommended reading below and other textbooks, outline the aetiology, presenting symptoms and treatment for selected diagnoses of cancer as they arise in your clinical setting (for example, lymphomas and sarcomas).
2. Investigate the prognosis and different stages of disease using resources available to you (for example, textbooks and fellow health care professionals). Take this a stage further and look at clients' expectations of the oncology and palliative care services.
3. Consider the occupational therapy that would be required in the acute stages of different treatments given the side effects described, bearing in mind that these side effects can be temporary, transitory or chronic in different individuals.

References

Beresford S (1995) Cancer. In Turner A (Ed) Occupational Therapy and Physical Dysfunction. 4th edn. Edinburgh: Churchill Livingstone, pp 823–4.
Chamberlain J (1988) Screening for early detection of cancer. In Prichard P (Ed) Oncology for Nurses and Health Care Professionals, Volume 1. London: Harper & Row.

Copp K (1989) Nursing patients having radiotherapy. In Borley D (Ed) Oncology for Nurses and Health Care Professionals, Volume 3. London: Harper & Row.

Duchesne G, Horwich A (1988) The nature of radiotherapy. In Prichard P (Ed) Oncology for Nurses and Health Care Professionals, Volume 1. London: Harper & Row.

Fredette S (1983) Evaluation of a Community Based Education Programme for Cancer Patients (Dissertation). Amherst, Massachusetts: University of Massachusetts.

Fredette S, Beattie H (1986) Living with cancer. A patient education program. Cancer Nursing 9(6): 308–16.

Gowing N, Fisher C (1988) The general pathology of tumours. In Pritchard P (Ed) Oncology for Nurses and Health Care Professionals, Volume 1. London: Harper & Row.

Hanratty JF, Higginson I (1994) Palliative Care in Terminal Illness. Oxford: Radcliffe Medical Press.

Milliken S, Lakhani A, Powles R (1988) Bone marrow transplantation. In Pritchard P (Ed) (1989) Oncology for Nurses and Health Care Professionals, Volume 1. London: Harper & Row.

Souhami R, Tobias J (1995) Cancer and its Management. Oxford: Blackwell.

Speechley V (1988) Nursing patients having chemotherapy. In Borley D (Ed) Oncology and Health Care Professionals, Volume 3, Chapter 3. London: Harper & Row.

Tobias J (1995) Cancer. What Every Patient Needs to Know. London: Bloomsbury.

Watson M, Ramirez A (1991) Cancer and Stress. Chichester: Wiley.

Westbury G (1988) Surgical oncology. In Pritchard R (Ed) Oncology for Nurses and Health Care Professionals, Volume 1. London: Harper & Row.

Recommended reading

Bennett S, Hill G, Trevan-Hawke J (1990) Occupational therapy in adult bone marrow transplantation. British Journal of Occupational Therapy 53(3): 101–4.

Cancer Research Campaign (1995) Factsheets. London: CRC.

Holmes S (1988) Radiotherapy. The Lisa Sainsbury Foundation Series. Reading: Austen Cornish.

Holmes S (1990) Cancer Chemotherapy. The Lisa Sainsbury Foundation Series. Reading: Austen Cornish.

Kaye P (1994) A–Z of Hospice and Palliative Medicine. Northampton, UK: EPL Publications.

McKay J, Hirano N (1994) The Chemotherapy Survival Guide. Oakland, USA: New Harbinger.

Patient Information Series (1996) London: The Royal Marsden NHS Trust.

Tobias J (1995) Cancers: What every patient needs to know. London: Bloomsbury.

Chapter 2
Dilemmas faced by Occupational Therapists in Oncology and Palliative Care

Jill Cooper

Occupational therapists, like all who work with dying clients and their families, are subject to a considerable amount of stress (Bennett, 1991). Tigges and Marcil (1988) state that

> [t]raditionally success in Occupational Therapy has been measured in terms of maintaining and increasing function so death of a patient appears to be in conflict with the life-saving goals of hospitals and with the aim of improving function.

Faulkner and Maguire (1994) look at the psychological cost of caring for cancer patients. They argue that, although the prime consideration in cancer care is the client, health carers may not be able to keep working in this field if they do not consider their own needs. In particular, it is important that the health professional should accept that care can be of good quality and can be effective without necessarily leading to a cure.

Each occupational therapist should consider why he or she wants to work with cancer or in palliative care. In particular, they should consider:

- 'Is it to fulfil a personal need?'
- 'Is it because I want to be adored by my clients and others?'
- 'What do I put into it and what do I get out?'
- 'Which areas do I personally find most stressful?'
- 'Am I able to deal with these?'

The occupational therapist needs to be aware of potential areas of stress. These include:

- lack of insight into one's own needs;
- caseload management and its pitfalls;
- breaking bad news;
- communication;
- conflict;
- grief;
- loss;
- cultural issues;
- spirituality;
- prioritization.

Insight into one's own needs

Revd Tom Gordon (1995) discussed issues for health care professionals dealing with bereavement. His advice included the following points:

- Be aware of your own feelings. You may be sad, or even angry, as you empathize with the bereaved. That's OK. But remember, you have to deal with your own feelings too and keep yourself healthy.
- Recognize your own sense of inadequacy. You don't have all the answers and you are not expected to have all the answers. Don't try too hard.
- Be in touch with your own parenting instincts. You will want to make the pain go away, to make it better by your loving and caring. You can't!
- Remember that not all questions have answers. Life and death are a mystery. Perhaps helping the bereaved to ask the right questions can be your gift to them.
- Don't ignore the death. It has happened. Pretending otherwise only puts off dealing with it.
- Be practical and share your time. One helpful action is worth a thousand clever words. A little of your time might be all that is needed.
- Be ready to listen. Allow the bereaved time and space to tell their story, or express their anger.
- Remember the uniqueness of grief. Every person has the right to react in his or her own way.
- Remember that grieving takes time. You can't rush adapting to change.

- Coax, but don't bully. Remember the thin dividing line between the two.
- Urge patience. Be careful to watch the platitudes.
- Be alert. Notice signs of deterioration and improvement.
- Don't slink away. Everyone else will.
- Remember that professional help may be needed in the end.

The last point can become a problem if the health care professional has insufficient support to deal with the difficulties that arise.

Faulkner and Maguire (1994) list some factors that influence whether or not staff cope:

- Personal awareness of the job.
- Balance between work and social life.
- Preparedness for the job being carried out.
- Organizational issues relating to management.
- Availability of support. If the necessary support is lacking, this will increase stress.
- Willingness to make use of support when it is offered.
- Ability to control working hours. Aspects of the job such as writing up notes should be carried out in normal working hours and work should not be allowed to accumulate.
- Taking a break when it is needed.
- Ability to devise one's own personal stress-management strategies. These include the ability to recognize when one is becoming tired and snappy and to look at what is going wrong.

Caseload management and pitfalls

Time management

The occupational therapist needs to organize the available working hours realistically, to vary the type and amount of client contact, to make a clear distinction between work and personal life, and to look after his or her own health and leisure needs (Gamage, McMahon and Shanahan, 1976). No occupational therapist can take on an infinite amount of work.

Section 3.1.2 of the UK Code of Ethics and Professional Conduct for Occupational Therapists reads as follows:

> Subject to any legal requirements to provide a minimum service, if the basic standards of treatment or intervention cannot be met at any time, for whatever reason, Occupational Therapists should decline to accept a referral or to initiate treatment.

Supervision

It is easy not to take advantage of supervision when it is available. Often, direct supervision may not be available as many occupational therapists work in isolation. It is therefore important that they receive support from other colleagues. It can be constructive for team members to present case studies to other team members and use peer-group feedback for support. Occupational therapists who are not being directly supervised should try to talk problems through with trust, confidentiality and objectivity. They should try to have a set session for feedback and discussion.

Debriefing sessions can be very supportive as they give the occupational therapist the opportunity to reflect on how circumstances were handled. They also allow those giving support or feedback to discuss alternative options and to consider how the occupational therapist feels.

Exposure to loss and bereavement needs to be acknowledged by the occupational therapist in order for him or her to deal with its cumulative effects. Individuals cope with loss, and react to it, in different ways. It does not necessarily demand additional resources, but the supervisor needs to be aware of, and sensitive to, staff needs in this respect.

Note-writing

It can be easy to neglect note-writing whilst trying to fulfil the requirements of service provision. This can become a source of stress. Notes must be written up regularly. Time should be set aside for this and adhered to strictly. There is a legal requirement to keep occupational therapy records up-to-date and documentation should be audited regularly as part of the service review.

Section 3.4 of the UK Code of Ethics and Professional Conduct for Occupational Therapists states that:

> Occupational Therapists shall accurately record all information related to professional activities.
>
> . . . Accurate, legible, factual and contemporaneous records and reports of occupational therapy intervention must be kept in order to provide information for professional colleagues and for legal purposes, such as client access and court reports.

Each department or service should have its own policy regarding the acceptable standard of note-keeping.

Breaking bad news

Whether clients are in the acute or palliative stages of cancer, the occupational therapist can still enable them to achieve some degree of mastery of self and the disease process, even when life expectancy may be limited (Lloyd, 1989).

Although the occupational therapist rarely has to break any bad news regarding diagnosis and prognosis, it may be necessary to do so when discussing, for example, prospects of walking again for those with spinal cord compression, or functional use of the arm as in brachial plexus problems or lymphoedema. The occupational thera-pist should not comment on the medical situation even when pressed by anxious relatives and should refer them to the medical practi-tioner. The simplest response is to explain that the purpose of occu-pational therapy sessions, together with the input from the rest of the multidisciplinary team, is to achieve optimum independence.

Occupational therapists should not remove hope from the client and carers, but they should stress that it is not possible to promise anything. They should suggest that clients take rehabilitation one step at a time and concentrate on the present – coping with the disability as it is now.

Emphasis should be placed on the enabling and positive aspects of equipment. This can help to counter the client's feeling of depen-dence and negativity. The introduction of a wheelchair, for example, facilitates some independence and control, and provides the first stage of rehabilitative gain. The occupational therapist can focus on each stage as it arises. The ultimate aim may be to progress to walk-ing. If independent mobility is not achieved then the client and carers can take as long as is needed to come to terms with this whilst still progressing with wheelchair mobility.

Kaye (1994) suggests that clients require:

- the correct amount of information; and
- the opportunity to talk and think about their situation.

He explains that communicating bad news is important to maintain trust, reduce uncertainty and prevent inappropriate hope which can lead to despair and waste precious time. This will facilitate the client's acceptance, enabling realistic plans to be made for the future.

Each individual's problems need to be addressed in a unique way. If the client's family is trying to protect him or her from knowing unpleasant facts then the multidisciplinary team should have a consistent approach to keep all the members informed. Most centres have a policy that, should the clients ask about their condition, they should be fully informed and the staff should not allow themselves to be manipulated by the family or carers. Kaye recommends asking the family 'what if the client asks to know?' and asking each family member what his or her understanding is of the disease and the situation. Opening up the conversation and creating an atmosphere of honesty and trust enables a frank exchange of worries and fears. Occupational therapists can then explain their role and how they can assist. With the whole team's support and input, the grieving process can begin and positive use can be made of the remaining time.

The Lisa Sainsbury Foundation have produced an excellent video, *The Dying Patient – Trying to Tell,* which explores how healthcare professionals approach imparting bad news and dealing with subsequent clinical appointments.

Communication

Communication aims to reduce uncertainty, encourage good working relationships and give the client and carers a positive direction in which to move.

Non-verbal communication is also essential when working with clients with cancer or receiving palliative care. This includes facial expression, eye contact, posture, body language, pitch and pace of voice, touch.

Confucius is reported to have said:

> If language is not correct, then what is said is not what is meant; if what is said is not what is meant, then what ought to be done remains undone.

Occupational therapists could ask themselves:

- 'Do we hide behind jargon?'
- 'If so, is it to protect ourselves because we manage to prevent the client asking difficult questions?'
- 'Is it to appear more knowledgeable and blind them with science?'

As clients become increasingly aware of their rights under the UK Patient's Charter, occupational therapists might be aware of being challenged more often about the content of treatment programmes. Occupational therapists have often been asked about their role by colleagues and the public alike. It is relatively easy to explain why a particular treatment medium or piece of equipment is chosen and it is important to respect the individual's right to question what is being done. Once clients know the reason for something they are more likely to be compliant and the treatment can be more successful –

particularly as the task of the occupational therapist is to enable and facilitate their independence.

The Royal Marsden Hospital has produced a series of patient information booklets on virtually all areas of treatment and disease for clients and carers.

Many occupational therapy departments produce information sheets on topics such as energy conservation and joint protection, and clients find these reassuring as they can refer back to them. Handouts regarding cancer and occupational therapy should only be distributed in conjunction with a treatment session. *It is important* they are not just handed out instead of an assessment and without professional support as there must be someone available to answer the questions that will arise from this information.

Brewin (1991) and Maguire (1983) suggest that there are no rules about the choice of words, facial expressions or tone of voice. These authors offer the following list of recommendations for conducting interviews:

DO

- allow time;
- ensure privacy;
- respect confidentiality;
- let the patient talk;
- listen to what the patient says;
- be sensitive to 'non-verbal cues' such as facial expression;
- gauge the need for information on an individual basis;
- permit painful topics;
- permit silences;
- unless an especially close rapport has been established, a sense of humour has to be used very delicately.

DON'T

- assume you know what is troubling the client;
- give false reassurance;
- overload the client with information;
- feel obliged to keep talking all the time;
- withhold information;
- tell lies;
- criticize or make judgements;
- give direct advice about psychological matters.

It is relatively rare in oncology centres or hospices for complete denial to take place or for clients not to know what is wrong. In the vast majority of centres, the policy is to keep the patient informed of diagnosis, progress and prognosis. If in doubt, ask the client about his or her understanding of the illness.

Conflict

Conflict may arise when an occupational therapist is not meeting the expectations of the team and/or the client. Occupational therapists have to clearly identify aims and objectives for treatment but they must also realize that they may be the focus of anger if the whole situation is becoming frustrating and unsatisfactory.

For example, suppose that, on a pre-discharge home assessment, the occupational therapist visits the home with the client from hospital. The wife specifically requests an item of equipment and focuses on this angrily, strongly declining other help that the health care professionals feel will be necessary (e.g. from a district nurse). Once the piece of equipment is provided, another problem arises and the occupational therapist becomes the focus of this. The basic problem is unresolved anger and denial at the diagnosis and the occupational therapist is simply in the line of fire. The multidisciplinary team, therefore, needs a consistent approach so as not to be sidetracked and to ensure that the real issues are addressed.

Conflict can be an energizing and vitalizing force if properly managed. It can have both positive and negative outcomes as it allows expression of worries and concerns and creates an opportunity for problems to be resolved. It has to be accepted that conflict is an inevitable feature of life in complex organizations and may occur at personal, interpersonal and group levels. If handled correctly, it can be contained and channelled positively. Ways in which conflict can be resolved include compromise, in which the parties involved decide on a solution by 'give and take', solving the underlying problem or avoiding it altogether.

Conflict can be linked to aggression, which can take the form of disagreement, anger, verbal abuse or violence. Different interventions are needed for diffusing and handling aggression as particular situations arise. Often, the client or carers need the opportunity to express their feelings – they need to be allowed to be angry in a safe environment and it is important to listen to them rather than shout them down. An empathetic approach will often help to diffuse the situation, not by identifying with them ('I know how you feel') but by acknowledging that it is understandable that they are angry and talking through the situation.

Aggression is a means of gaining power over others. Clients and carers are in the position of having lost control over their lives because of the disease and impairment and so they need to have some autonomy over decisions and help. A client may not want a whole string of different health care professionals coming in and out of his or her house. Compromise is therefore necessary in order to maintain the client safely without taking over.

Occupational therapists might consider who they work with and against in their work setting. For example, an occupational therapist might work well with clients, carers and multidisciplinary staff but might come into conflict with budget holders over the provision of service. He or she might then be able to examine what can be resolved.

Suppose the occupational therapist visits a young client with a life-threatening illness, and the mother will not let him or her talk to the client but instead berates the entire service and tells the occupational therapist what is needed. The occupational therapist needs to consider:

* confidentiality, how much the mother knows;
* boundary-setting, making it clear what the occupational therapist's role is;
* allowing the mother to express concerns and anger then calmly addressing the issues;
* asking the mother what she wants for her child;
* explaining that the occupational therapist is ultimately working for the client;
* giving back control to the family and facilitating a situation where they work together to accept the multidisciplinary team and service's input.

Lanciotti and Hopkins (1995) advise the following proactive principles when dealing with hostility:

* recognize early warning signs;
* use reason and be reasonable;
* relate;
* reply to the underlying emotion;
* retreat – this is entirely appropriate and permissible;
* respond and react;

- report;
- record;
- review and re-examine.

If the occupational therapist becomes involved in a conflict situation, he or she should reflect on the reasons for the conflict. This should be done either with formal supervision or informal support.

Loss

Loss can take many forms: it can involve loss of a job, loss of aspirations, of home and security, of children, of a partner (in death or divorce), of a body part or loss of self-esteem, independence, friends, health or time. Losses are multifaceted; loss of mobility alone can lead to changes in:

Role	Social relationships, work
Physical integrity	Body image
Mental integrity	Weight changes
Hair loss	Unfamiliar emotions and behaviour.
Independence	Self-esteem
Dignity	Sexual function
Faith	Bodily function
Life expectancy	Hopes
Autonomy	Freedom
Comfort	Dreams
Privacy	

Most health care professionals are likely to be the focus of the client's feelings of loss at one time or another. Occupational therapists typically find that they are blamed when there is a delay in the provision of equipment. Equipment is a tangible item on which people can focus their feelings of loss. There is a danger here of transference of hopelessness from the client, carer or colleagues to the therapist. Occupational therapists need to be aware of this but they should be able to recognize their own feelings and those of the client.

Having said this, non-provision of equipment can lead to delayed discharge from hospital. It is a vital part of the occupational therapy programme to anticipate problems and not end up mopping up a crisis. With increased demand for resources and decreased funding, occupational therapists need to be aware of this potential cause of stress.

Grief

Although there are observable and well-documented patterns of grief, there is no such thing as a 'normal time span for grief'. This can be very distressing and even annoying to relatives and friends who may think that 'it is time he got over it'. The grieving process could well commence prior to death. The client and carers may grieve for loss of function (mobility, body image and role) as well as loss of life.

Grief is a 'normal' psychological response to any significant loss and there is no correct reaction for health care professionals. It depends on the individual. Occupational therapists can play a role in supporting the client, carers and each other by helping them adjust to loss in their own way. Figure 2.1 shows the stages that people may go through.

Occupational therapists have counselling skills and techniques that are used within this area of work. However, within most units there will be other members of the multidisciplinary team who are employed as counsellors and they have more extensive training in this field. Occupational therapists can use their skills to recognize the need for referral to other agencies and they should not counsel clients with cancer.

Simple techniques can be used to build a rapport with clients and to encourage them to express themselves more openly so that the occupational therapist can assess whether counselling is necessary. These include the following:

- *Avoiding closed questions* (questions that can be answered monosyllabically with 'yes' or 'no'). This can be done by using words like 'what', 'where', 'when', 'why' or 'who'. For example, the question 'Did the doctor tell you about your illness?' can be changed to 'What/how much did the doctor tell you about your illness?'
- *Reflection* – mirroring and repeating key points of conversation to clarify them and to encourage the client to continue speaking. For example, suppose a middle-aged man recovering from an amputation says: 'I'll never get used to this. Sometimes I think I would have been better off if I'd died. What's the point of living when you are a cripple?' The response might be 'So you feel you'll never get used to your amputation, that you sometimes think you'd have been better off dying, and you wonder what the point of living is?' Mirroring, reflecting and clarifying enables the occupational therapist to check that he or she has understood clients' words correctly before encouraging them to share their concerns.

	DENIAL	DEVELOPING AWARENESS	RESOLUTION
	Death of spouse up to 2 weeks	2 weeks –2 years	2 years –5 years
Physical reactions	Shock	Loss of vitality. Physical symptoms of stress. Irrational behaviour – often coming in waves lasting 20–60 minutes. Psychosomatic illness, often parallels symptoms of deceased (may not be reversed)	
Emotional	Numbness Cottonwool feeling Denial	Outbursts of grief (pining, crying, exhaustion) Depression or sadness Anger - against deceased, medicine, God ("why?") Loss of confidence and self-approval Guilt ('if only . . .?') Loneliness – especially in older bereaved Idealising of the deceased	**Resolution** 1 The resolve that one will cope 2 Sense of detachment allowing freedom of action 3 Feeling it is now OK to enjoy social contacts etc.
External factors affecting behaviour	Circumstances of death and funeral arrangements Family Religious beliefs and culture	Financial loss or gain Loss of status Anniversaries Society's disapproval of overt emotion and avoidance of death	Acceptance of new status by society. Role of organizations such as: Cruse Society for Compassionate Friends

From *Letting Go* by Ian Ainsworth-Smith and Peter Speck

Figure 2.1: 'Normal' patterns of bereavement behaviour

Cultural issues

Spector (1991) feels it is often difficult to establish whether a person's beliefs are founded in religion or ethnic and cultural heritage. Ian Ainsworth-Smith (1996) writes:

> Spiritual care has often been in the past delegated to 'official' chaplains or religious representatives; alternatively it may be studiously avoided by staff who may feel inadequate because of their own lack of formal belief.

Health care professionals should acquire background knowledge about how disease is viewed within specific communities and about what determines people's individuality and status within various cultural hierarchies. Our society is becoming increasingly multicultural and there is a growing need for greater understanding of the various ethnic and religious groups that make up the community. This does not mean that one should hold any particular religious views oneself but one should respect the needs of the client. Neuberger (1987) has pointed out that it makes all the difference to someone in strange surroundings, often in pain and discomfort, to have something familiar such as a Koran and a prayer mat.

The health care professional must not, however, assume that someone of a different culture is, for example, a devout Moslem or Hindu. Clients might not want religious traditions imposed on them. The occupational therapist should establish whether the client is practising any religion at the very outset of treatment. Should food restrictions, dress code or prohibition of participation in dressing assessment be an issue, then the occupational therapist needs to find out what the patient will and will not do, both in a domestic setting and in treatment sessions. The family or a religious adviser might also be able to advise about what the client is able to do. Difficulties are unlikely to arise if one is honest and says 'you tell me what is and is not permitted' and if one shows genuine respect and interest in the client's culture.

Kubler-Ross (1969) discusses the trend towards training health care professionals – particularly medical students – to make scientific and technical achievements and the demise of interpersonal contact. She points out that they learn to prolong life but receive little training in the meaning of life, or how to communicate effectively with patients.

Illness might affect how clients' communities view and accept them. Within certain cultural groups, body-image alteration and dysfunction can affect an individual's standing within the family, the community, at work and within the religious community. It could even lead to exclusion from worship in a holy place. Specific difficulties arise with hair loss, amputation of body parts (such as a limb or breast) and stoma.

Helman (1992) states that concepts surrounding the idea of body image may be divided into three categories:

- Beliefs about the optimal shape and size of the body including clothing and surface decoration.
- Beliefs about the inner structure of the body.
- Beliefs about how the body functions.

Hair loss

Noyes (1988) writes that

> Hair throughout the centuries has had powerful influences on individuals and society. It has meant strength, power, politics, wealth and beauty.

Hair loss is common among Western males and is associated with the ageing process. For women it is perceived as far more damaging and is a clear indication to others of a serious illness. Although there are wigs, turbans or scarves available, and these can be acceptable to some, hair loss can be emotionally devastating as styling, colour and length make social statements about the individual.

Other societies place far greater emphasis on hair and hair loss. Amongst some Cantonese-speaking communities, hair is a symbol of power to absorb life forces and a medium for losing toxins and impurities that arise from disease and from the death of a family member. Hair loss leads to fears regarding an individual's ability to recover from illness.

The Sikh faith views the intactness of the body as extremely important and hair loss diminishes both men and women. In African cultures hair loss can be an outward sign of loss of fertility. Rastafarians, in particular, see dreadlocks as symbols of black dignity and inward power so loss of hair may be devastating to their self-image. Orthodox Jewish women customarily have short hair or a shorn head whereas most Jewish women value their hair. The more strict Christian faiths such as the Amish, the Taylorites and the Exclusive Brethren wear their hair long as a sign of God's favour.

Breast loss due to mastectomy

As well as feelings of loss of sexuality there may be shame associated with loss of a breast due to feelings of a lack of self-worth influenced by culture and religion. Western society values the breast shape and size. Altered body shape certainly affects women's feelings of self-confidence and how others view them. In Chinese folk medicine, breast milk was felt to provide immunity to the infant.

Stomas

Colostomies, ileostomies and urostomies may not only threaten the individual's self-esteem and body image but may alter his or her ability to worship. This can lead to ostracism and may be viewed as uncleanliness. The Islamic faith does not allow ablutions during prayer and, as stomas cannot be controlled voluntarily, an individual may need to leave and start prayers again after each wash. Occupational therapists should be aware of the implications of culture on such fundamental tasks.

Spirituality

Occupational therapists often claim to adopt an holistic approach to care. This holistic approach needs to incorporate spirituality. Spirituality is not the exclusive domain of any professional body but is an issue that should be addressed by all team members.

Each religion contains various denominations and different cultures contain various subcultures. There is thus a danger that unwarranted assumptions might be made about the client's needs because of one's own limited understanding of a particular faith or community. The chaplaincy should be able to advise on support for any faith.

Setting individual religions aside, occupational therapy assists clients and carers in spiritual matters by helping them set goals and priorities. By doing this, the occupational therapist enables clients to see the purpose in what they are doing and to identify what is important to them.

Helfrich and Kielhofner (1994) advised:

> Occupational Therapy can only transform lives if patients see meaning and relevance to their own life stories. The task of Occupational Therapy is to become an episode in the patient's narrative.

Occupational therapists work with and for their clients and so become a part of their narratives, a part of their rehabilitation process and their adaptation to their present lifestyle (Mattingly, 1991).

Stoter (1996) describes how, although religion is a component of spiritual care, there are many other aspects of spirituality. In particular, allowing clients to express themselves is fundamental to the occupational therapy process in all areas of treatment, from activities of daily living to reminiscence therapy. It has the following effects:

- it increases self-esteem by allowing clients to reflect on what they have achieved;
- it enables clients to emphasize their individuality at a time when they may be losing their own identity due to frequent hospital appointments, hospital admissions and gradual institutionalization;
- it strengthens their identity as productive individuals;
- it gives them the opportunity to share life experiences with others, so helping them see the client in his or her former roles in life;
- it enables them to undertake the transition from one role to another;
- it helps them to accept the stage of life at which they find themselves;
- it encourages them to air their concerns;
- it helps the problem-solving process by enabling others to identify what the specific problems are;
- it allows the occupational therapist to help the client to turn negative thoughts into positive thoughts;
- it help clients provide meaning, a sense of fulfilment and purpose to their lives.

Occupational therapists can look at what clients wish to gain from their remaining time. If one allows clients to discuss aspects of their life history, rather than just asking them to give a medical history, 'such accounts may help to fit the pieces together, to draw conclusions, and to give continuity to the story so that it remains a comprehensible whole' (Kirsh, 1996).

Sharing one's feelings helps one to 'connect' with others; one makes one's time, space and feelings available for others.

Egan and Delaat (1994) discuss how illness can create a block to spiritual expression and how examining one's values and beliefs may cause a spiritual crisis. Illness often causes a change in life roles; sometimes this involves either a permanent or a temporary loss of roles. This, in turn, may result in clients no longer being 'connected' with themselves or with others because of reduced self-esteem. It may cause them to question their place in life and the meaning and purpose of what they are doing.

Miller (1990) gives guidelines for assisting an individual through crisis:

- first normalize the crisis;
- affirm the individual's strengths;

- recognize and respect the individual's subjective experiences;
- balance these experiences with the outer world;
- convey hope and acceptance.

By giving practical help, reassurance, advice and support, the occupational therapist can help the client regain some control. By listening with unconditional positive regard, the occupational therapist can provide great support.

In order to listen carefully, the occupational therapist needs to reflect on his or her own values. Kirsch (1996) discusses ways of looking at the 'meaning and purpose of one's life' and how this influences performance and everyday occupational therapy practice. Being aware of one's own spirituality, exploring one's own values and incorporating this understanding into supervision or support can help in accepting others' responses. It is easy to be uncomfortable with clients' feelings being 'unloaded' and Egan and Delaat (1994) suggest one should take time to consider:

- What makes life meaningful for you from moment to moment?
- Whom do you connect with and how do you do this?
- How does this enrich your life?
- What sense do you make out of the pain and suffering that you view each day?
- Where do you see beauty in the world?
- How do these things fit in with your own religious belief?
- What questions remain for you?

Any response from the occupational therapist needs to encourage further discussion from the client. It should not involve the occupational therapist imposing his or her own opinions.

Occupational therapy will not necessarily make a client more healthy but intervention allows expression and adaptation to dysfunction. Bathing aids, for example, do not aid spirituality but they allow choice and control and enable clients to carry out activities that are important to them.

Muldoon and King (1991) write that the basic dignity and worth of all individuals and the recognition of a drive to growth inherent in all individuals are two important aspects of spirituality. By promoting, encouraging and facilitating everyday activities of daily living and a means of expression, the occupational therapist helps clients to achieve both.

Summary

This chapter has touched briefly on some of the issues faced during the working day. Given the nature of some of these issues it is not surprising that occupational therapists are subject to stress. In order to deal with this, they have to appreciate the subtle pressures involved and must take action if they find it is all becoming too much for them. If the sheer volume of work becomes too great, this has to be analysed; work must be prioritized and a decision has to be made about what can be managed.

A list of care priorities can be used to identify which areas take precedence. Such a list is provided in Appendix 1A.

Occupational therapists working in oncology and palliative care need to be aware of key points in coping with working with clients with a limited life span. These are:

- support;
- teamwork;
- prioritization;
- realistic aims and objectives;
- understanding and respect of patients, carers and fellow colleagues needs;
- acknowledging one's own limitations and knowing when to refer.

Action points

1. Do you feel that your role is clearly understood by colleagues in other professions? If not, how would you promote your role in a positive and dynamic way?
2. Do you find your job leaves you tired and dissatisfied? How would you identify why this is happening? Which areas could realistically be improved in the short term and the long term?
3. Does the occupational therapist in oncology and palliative care receive sufficient support in the work setting? What support mechanisms could be sought or arranged? From which colleagues?

References

Ainsworth-Smith I, Speck P (1982) Letting Go. London: SPCK Holy Trinity Church.
Ainsworth-Smith I (1986) Foreword. In Neuberger J, Caring for Dying People of Different Faiths. Reading: Austen Cornish.
Barraclough J (1994) Cancer and Emotion. Chichester: Wiley.

Bennett S (1991) Issues confronting occupational therapists working with terminally ill patients. British Journal of Occupational Therapy 54(1): 8–10.

Bernard P (1991) Beyond burnout. Nursing Standard 5(43): 46–8.

Brewin TB (1991) Three ways of giving bad news. Lancet 337: 1207–9.

Canadian Association of Occupational Therapists (1991) Occupational Therapy Guidelines for Client-Centred Practice. Toronto: CAOT Publications.

College of Occupational Therapists (1990) Statement on Guidelines for Documentation. London: College of Occupational Therapists.

College of Occupational Therapists (1990) Statement on Supervision in Occupational Therapy. London: College of Occupational Therapists.

College of Occupational Therapists (1995) Code of Ethics and Professional Conduct for Occupational Therapists. London: College of Occupational Therapists.

Comaroff J (1982) Medicine, symbol and ideology. In Wright P and Treacher A (Eds) The Problem of Medical Knowledge. Edinburgh: Edinburgh University Press.

Egan M, Delaat MD (1994) Considering spirituality in occupational therapy practice. Canadian Journal of Occupational Therapy 61(2): 95–101.

Faulkner A (1992) Effective Interaction with Patients. Edinburgh: Churchill Livingstone.

Faulkner A, Maguire P (1994) Talking to Cancer Patients and their Relatives. Oxford: Oxford Medical Publications.

Gamage SL, McMahon PS, Shanahan PM (1976) The occupational therapist and terminal illness. Learning to cope with death. American Journal of Occupational Therapy 30(5): 294–9.

Helfrich C, Kielhofner G (1994) Volitional narratives and the meaning of therapy. American Journal of Occupational Therapy 48: 319–26.

Helman C (1992) Culture, Health and Illness. London: Wright.

Kirsch B (1996) A narrative approach to addressing spirituality in occupational therapy: exploring personal meaning and purpose. Canadian Journal of Occupational Therapy 63(1): 55–61.

Kubler-Ross E (1969) On Death and Dying. London: Souvenir Press.

Lanciotti L, Hopkins A (1995) Breaking the cycle. Nursing Standard 10(11): 22–4.

Lloyd C (1989) Maximising occupational role performance with terminally ill patients. British Journal of Occupational Therapy 52(6): 227–9.

Maguire P, Brooke M, Tait A, Thomas C, Sellwood R (1983) The effect of counselling on physical disability and social recovery after mastectomy. Clinical Oncology 9: 319–24.

Maslach C (1981) Burnout: The Cost of Caring. Englewood Cliffs, New Jersey: Prentice Hall.

Mattingly C (1991) The narrative nature of clinical reasoning. American Journal of Occupational Therapy 45: 998–1005.

Miller JS (1990) Mental illness and spiritual crisis: implications for psychiatric rehabilitation. Psychosocial Rehabilitation Journal 14(2): 29–47.

Mischler E (1986) The Discourse of Medicine. Cambridge, Massachussetts: Harvard University Press.

Muldoon M, King JN (1991) A spirituality for the long haul: response to chronic illness. Journal of Religion and Health 30: 99–108.

Neuberger J (1987) Caring for Dying People of Different Faiths. Reading: Austen Cornish.

Noyes, DD (1988) Beauty and Cancer. Los Angeles: AC Press.

Spector R (1985) Cultural Diversity in Health and Illness. New York: Appleton & Lange.

Stoter D (1996) In Penson J, Fisher R (Eds) Palliative Care for People with Cancer, Chapter 11. London: Edward Arnold.

Tigges KN, Marcil WM (1988) Terminal and Life Threatening Illness: an Occupational Behaviour Perspective. Thorofare, NJ: Slack.

Recommended reading

Clark D (Ed) (1993) The Future for Palliative Care. Buckingham: Open University Press.

Dickensen D, Johnson M (Eds) (1993) Death, Dying and Bereavement. London: Sage Press.

Helman C (1992) Culture, Health and Illness. London: Wright.

Kaye P (1995) Breaking Bad News. Northampton, UK: EPL Publications.

Lindenfield G (1993) Managing Anger: Positive Strategies for Dealing with Difficult Emotions. London: Thorsons.

Lupton D (1994) Medicine as Culture. London: Sage Press.

Neuberger J and White J (1991) A Necessary End. London: Papermac.

Penson J, Fisher R (1995) Palliative Care for People with Cancer. London: Edward Arnold.

Rubin, T (1969) The Angry Book. London: Collier Macmillan.

Chapter 3
Principles of
Occupational
Therapy
Intervention

Jill Cooper

Occupational therapy intervention with the client in an oncology or palliative care setting includes:

- an appreciation of the client's difficulties;
- establishing rapport;
- the initial interview;
- informing and enabling the client;
- provision of service;
- facilitating and enabling optimum functional independence.

Unless the occupational therapist is working in a purely oncology setting it is likely that the referral to occupational therapy will only be made when a severe functional difficulty arises. Even if the client is not seen in the acute stages, it is important for the occupational therapist to know what the client may be experiencing. Being faced with a cancer or palliative care client is often a worrying experience for any health care professional. However, what is important is not the illness with which the client has been diagnosed but rather the difficulties that client is experiencing. Occupational therapists may not be experts in cancer or palliative care but they are experts in occupational therapy, the occupational therapy process and the occupational therapy intervention. Core skills are based on a problem-solving approach.

This involves:

- gathering and analysing information following referral;
- assessing, defining and establishing the problem;

- prioritizing;
- planning and preparing for treatment;
- providing treatment;
- evaluating outcomes;
- continuation of treatment, discharging or reviewing.

Appreciation of clients' difficulties

Hagopian (1993) describes some issues that commonly face patients:

- Cognitive adaptation: appraising the threat. This involves coping with illness and its effects, managing the hospital environment, the tests, treatment, symptoms and exposure to possibly dozens of health care professionals. The individual needs to cope with appearing fairly well as friends, family and colleagues may have different expectations of how one should look. He or she also has to appraise what is happening and continue to reappraise the situation as coping mechanisms are developed.
- Vulnerability. Clients often say that they feel that control has been taken away from them and that they need to share their concerns. This is where all the staff need to show that they care and inspire confidence by their expertise.
- Denial. This defence mechanism might be used in order to escape from the realities. Complete denial is uncommon. Denial usually shows itself at different levels such as not believing results and putting discomfort down to other reasons.
- Attribution: the search for meaning. Clients will want to find reasons for the disease, attributing it to stress, environmental pollution, familial patterns.
- Downward comparison: 'it could have been worse'. People often compare themselves to others who are less fortunate in an effort to be positive.
- Reappraisal of life: a second look at values. The diagnosis of cancer frequently causes people to reassess their values, attitudes, beliefs and priorities.
- A sense of mastery. Gaining control. Different mechanisms, such as changing diet, practising self-hypnosis or using imagery, can be employed to enable clients to regain control over their own lives.
- Spirituality. Each individual encounters this issue in different ways. It may involve religion or spirituality in a more abstract sense. Clients might experience the need for spiritual support.

Intervention may be required at the following stages:

- denial;
- relapse/remission;
- recovery;
- the survival phase;
- the chronic, continuing and terminal phases.

The roles of the client are likely to change in the following respects:

- the client may take on the sick role;
- the carer may push the client into the sick role;
- the children may take on the adult role;
- the breadwinner and head of the family may now have leisure time which was not available previously;
- the client may have goals relating to the palliative stages of life to which he or she needs to adjust;
- the client loses autonomy and control of his or her own life;
- the client may be subjected to cultural influences concerning expected change in roles, including perceptions by other members of his or her family and community.

Changes in roles may occur subconsciously or as a coping mechanism.

In order to help the client, occupational therapists need to be confident of their own abilities at whatever stage they become involved. They must know what their core skills are and must apply them. They must also have a clear idea of what can be offered from the point of view of rehabilitation and equipment, but also being clear about what cannot be offered – knowing their limitations (again by identifying core skills).

Approaching a new client and establishing rapport

When approaching a client for the first time, the occupational therapist should:

- give his or her name and title (the occupational therapist should always wear a badge – the clients cannot be expected to remember everyone);
- simply state that the occupational therapist's job involves ensuring that the clients are managing as safely and comfortably at home as possible.

The following checklist should enable the occupational therapist to structure the initial interview and assessment:

Client's social situation:
Lives alone/lives with:
Accommodation:
Type:
Owned by:
Internal layout:
(access, internal steps/stairs, rooms downstairs/upstairs)
Current functional status:
Mobility:
Stairs:
Transfers:
Bed:
Chair:
Toilet:
Bath:
Personal ADL:
Domestic ADL:
Cognition/communication:
Plan:

Some of the details may already have been covered in the multidisciplinary care plan, so it is better just to ask the client to confirm them rather than asking him or her to repeat them again.

After the initial interview the client can be informed about what is available and how to obtain it. This might or might not involve a visit to the occupational therapy department. It is not the role of the occupational therapist to impose the service; he or she should, however, ensure that clients know what they can borrow, expect from social services, or purchase themselves.

Hens (1989) said:

Functional evaluation incorporates three inter-related processes . . .
  i)   assessment of functional status,
  ii) classification based on functional abilities,
  iii) evaluation of functional progress relative to time, therapeutic and other factors.

On occasions the occupational therapist may find that the client does not want to talk to him or her. The client may experience feelings of anger and frustration from the acute stages of a disease through to the later stages. Clients may be considering their own mortality; they may have just been faced with the results of investigations and tests, or they may been questioned endlessly by different professionals.

In the acute stage, the client may not be in a position to take on board a huge amount of information. If the newly diagnosed client is trying to call on his or her own coping skills to deal with what he or she is being told, the last thing that client wants is to be approached by yet another person asking questions and offering advice.

This is where a succinct written explanation of occupational therapy and what it can offer is of help. If the client does not want to know, then leave this explanation with a contact number. If the therapist is particularly worried about the client, he or she can always call back or contact the client later to ensure the client has not changed his or her mind.

It is important to listen to the clients' worries, note their problems and be aware of the individuals to whom matters outside the scope of occupational therapy might be referred (such as members of the medical team, clinical nurse specialists or the chaplaincy).

Problems encountered with surgery may involve:

- a need for information about how the body heals;
- a need for information about post-surgery complications;
- a need for information about exercises;
- allowing time for pain to subside;
- coping with disfigurement.

Problems encountered with chemotherapy and radiotherapy include:

- tiredness (combined chemotherapy and radiotherapy treatments are exhausting);
- emotional 'let down' once the treatment is finished as the client has developed a dependency on attending the hospital;
- side effects (described in Chapter 1);
- there may be problems with the amount of time taken for the benefits of treatment to be noticed – it can take up to three weeks before there is a noticeable improvement.

There are so many different things for clients to consider, so many choices, so much information and conflicting ideas, but the client must decide what treatment to choose. If the client is in a dilemma, he or she should write down his or her questions and worries so that they can be presented to the specialist at the clinic. Palliative care clients have limited time so do not waste it.

The provision of information is a positive way to inform and enable the client and to restore some autonomy. Upon calling back to check if anything is needed, the occupational therapist is likely to find:

- that clients may not require anything but are pleased to see the occupational therapist as they are 'too well to need you' – which is reassuring for them; or
- the occupational therapist may find a comprehensive shopping list has been drawn up by the client and/or carers.

Having raised clients' awareness of what is available, the occupational therapist needs to be ready with information as to where and how they can obtain everything (the social services, occupational therapy loans, private hire or purchase of equipment).

Providing service

Once needs are identified, the occupational therapist should arrange for provision of equipment and other interventions speedily. Each individual service needs to set its own procedure for the loan or provision of equipment. If the service is unable to provide equipment, it is extremely useful to have sheets printed with a selection of agencies where equipment might be obtained. An example of a hospital 'loan of equipment procedure' is given in Appendix 1B.

In order to obtain equipment or adaptations from Social Services in the UK a person must meet the service eligibility criteria for occupational therapy. A person must be registrable as a disabled person and must be permanently and substantially handicapped by illness, injury or congenital deformity as stated in Section 29(1) of the National Assistance Act 1948.

Resources

The following issues should be considered when assessing a particular piece of equipment:

- Does it suit the needs of the client?
- Does the client want it and will he or she use it?

- Does another health care professional want the client to have it and is the occupational therapist simply trying to keep that colleague happy?
- Have all the safety factors been considered?
- Is the occupational therapist supplying equipment as his or her way of coping/reacting to a hopeless and difficult situation?

When a client requires expensive resources such as a stairlift, the installation of a downstairs WC or a house extension, the request should be referred to social services early on. If the referral is received when the client is in the later stages of an illness, it may be less likely that a disabled facilities grant will be appropriate.

The disabled facilities grant (DFG)

The disabled facilities grant is available for a range of works needed to adapt a disabled person's home. It is available to people who are registered as disabled or those who could be registered and who are owner-occupiers or tenants, including council or housing association tenants. The grant is also available to landlords on behalf of tenants, or to individuals who live with a disabled person.

The DFG is mandatory for adaptations that are essential to give freedom of movement in and around the house. These could include:

- widening doors or installing a ramp for access to the house;
- improving access to the rooms by installing stair lift, ramps and hand rails;
- providing suitable bathrooms and kitchen facilities (for example, at wheelchair height);
- improving the heating system;
- adapting heating or lighting controls to make them easier to use;
- improving access in the house to allow the disabled person to care for dependants.

The DFG is discretionary for a wide range of other changes to the house to make it more suitable for the disabled person's accommodation, welfare or employment needs.

When a person applies for a grant, his or her need for the adaptation will be assessed by an occupational therapist from the Social Services Department, to check that the proposed work is necessary and appropriate to meet the person's needs and that it is practicable with respect to the condition of the property.

The amount of money granted in the DFG is assessed by means testing the individual's income and savings. Once an application for a DFG has been made, the local authority must give a decision within six months. It is important that no work is started before the grant has been confirmed in writing otherwise the grant is likely to be refused. People who are required to pay part of the cost of adaptations but who cannot afford this should discuss the issue with the Social Services Department to see whether any additional help is available. Help should be requested under the Chronically Sick and Disabled Persons Act or the Children Act (1974).

The length of time involved in setting up a DFG should not prevent applications from being made but it is only fair to advise clients of the realities concerning the resources available to them these days. If they wish to purchase equipment privately there should be no difficulty in providing addresses of reputable local dealers who can send their representatives and advisors. It is important to provide several contact names so as not to be seen as being biased. Such information can be obtained from local Disabled Living Centres.

Clients are entitled to be considered for a DFG regardless of their life expectancies. If they are referred and the application is rejected, however (perhaps due to means testing and/or prognosis), this means that valuable time has been lost – time in which the clients could have been using and benefiting from equipment or services purchased privately.

An alternative to making expensive alterations is arranging living accommodation on one level which may appear to be a less acceptable compromise but may, in the end, be the simplest option for the client.

Referrals for major adaptations may not always be realistic or viable and the occupational therapist has to use professional judgement in these cases.

Facilitating and enabling

Each service will have its own resources and therapists have their own preference for equipment. The occupational therapist can use problem-solving techniques to establish how functional difficulties concerning such matters as mobility, stairs, 'transfers' (the ability to transfer from one surface to another), activities of daily living, cognition and, more specifically, upper-limb dysfunction, clothing and dressing may be overcome.

Mobility

When the client has difficulties with mobility, referral to the physio-therapist is essential for assessment and appropriate intervention. This may involve daily walking practice as well as provision of a stick, crutches, a walking frame or a Rolator frame, and techniques/exercises to maximize muscle power and strength.

The occupational therapist can assess the need for, and request, strategically placed grab rails or additional bannister rails to facilitate improved transfers and safer walking up and down steps. Whether social services arrange for rails to be fitted depends on where the client lives. Guidelines for consideration when requesting these are set out in Equipment for Disabled People (1995). One of the main factors is to assess and analyse the client's dysfunction and to provide equipment to solve the problem (for example, the rail should be positioned to help the patient transfer safely and independently).

Ramps and steps are also covered in Equipment for Disabled People (1995). Installation of ramps may be necessary and it is vital to remember that the optimum gradient for a wheelchair ramp is 1:20. This would make the ramp very long so it may need to have a turn and a landing area. A gradient of 1:12 is the maximum recommended. The design, surface and materials of permanent ramps all have to be considered for safety and aesthetic appeal.

Referral should be made to the local social services occupational therapist for assessment and advice on provision. Temporary ramps can be loaned to enable access but safety factors must be considered to ensure that they fit securely on sloping or rough ground.

The occupational therapist may be called on to assess and provide a wheelchair if walking is not possible or if it is extremely limited due to weakness, shortness of breath, bony metastases, spinal cord compression or pain.

The purpose of the wheelchair should be identified:

- Is it for everyday use?
- Is it for occasional use (for example, for travelling to the shops)?
- Is it to be self-propelling?
- Is it to be pushed by an attendant?

Assessment and prescription will depend on local resources, including the results of an assessment of how long it will take to provide a wheelchair and on whether the occupational therapy service can loan one in the meantime.

Pressure care and prevention of pressure injuries are extremely important for the wheelchair user and must be emphasized to the client and carers. It is particularly important where the client has mobility problems. If a wheelchair is not being used for moving from one point to another but the client is simply sitting out in it, the client should be encouraged to transfer into and sit in an upholstered armchair which will provide better postural support than the canvas back and seat of a wheelchair. Seating accessories might include head and arm supports as well as lumbar and seating cushions.

Stairs

As discussed before, major installations such as stairlifts require expert advice from the occupational therapist. The main point to consider when assessing such installations is that the equipment fits the client's needs. It is vital to ensure that the lift takes the client to the top of the stairs and that it does not leave a step or two to be negotiated at the top or bottom. If a curved staircase is too complicated, a through-floor lift might be considered. The client needs to be aware that installation of such a lift is not suitable in accommodation where a pre-payment meter is in place: the money in the meter might run out when the stairlift is between floors. Various aspects of how lifts run need to be considered. Consideration should also be given to the various types of lift (seated, standing or wheelchair-platform).

In addition to the financial assessments required for the disabled facilities grant, specific points to be considered are:

- the client's level of mobility and dexterity in operating the controls and safety belt;
- the client's ability to travel safely sitting or standing alone;
- dysfunction (such as visual impairment, confusion, incontinence, pain, lack of sensation, pressure sores, contractures or limited range of joint movement);
- the suitability of the property for such an installation – particularly with respect to the stairway, headroom and landing;
- possible obstruction of passageways, doorways, access to cupboards;
- adequate light on stairways and landings at all times;
- sufficient leg and foot room in relation to where the platform stops by the wall.

Transfers

All employers in the United Kingdom are now obliged to provide moving and handling training and guidelines, and it is the employees' responsibility to familiarize themselves with the local employer's regulations and College of Occupational Therapists guidelines on the subject. The occupational therapist must attend annual training sessions.

The following excerpts from College of Occupational Therapists (1995) are important:

1. The Health and Safety at Work Act 1974 places a general duty on an employer 'to ensure, so far is reasonably practicable, the health, safety and welfare at work of all employees (Section 2(1)) . . .

Section One: Management Responsibilities.

1.2 Occupational Therapists handle inanimate loads and people, both of which produce handling risks. A code of practice should be developed which sets out safe approaches to manual handling . . .

Section Two: Implementation and Supervision.

2.3 All staff must ensure that they are professionally up to date and are competent handlers, particularly of consumers, and that they follow regulations (MHOR 92) and guidance notes . . .

Section Four: Information Needs.

4.1 Manual handling assessment is often provided by a multi-disciplinary team. Within this skill mix the specialist knowledge of the occupational therapist is paramount. Their two great contributions are the knowledge of manual handling equipment and the ergonomic approach to work . . .

Section Five: The Ergonomic Approach.

5.11 Where the handling assessment involves the participation of other staff or carers, a professional responsibility must be considered in involving handlers who are less than fit.

With all equipment, the simplest techniques are often the most effective and avoid unnecessary cluttering. For example, patient-handling slings are made of thick, moulded plastic. The handgrips have rounded edges and non-slip surfaces that are comfortable to hold. The sling is placed under the thighs to enable the helpers to keep their backs straight when lifting and carry out assisted standing transfers, as shown in Figure 3.1.

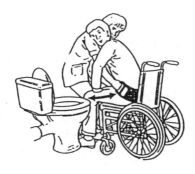

Figure 3.1: A patient-handling sling

In order to facilitate client's transfers, strategically placed grabrails can be of help, as illustrated in Figure 3.2.

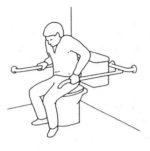

Pushing the body up

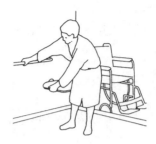

Pulling the body up

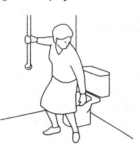

Steadying the body when it is being lowered

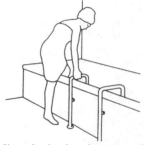

Steading the body when transferring from one position to another

Figure 3.2: Grabrails

Mobility within bed, in/out bed

Mobility and independence depend on the degree of disability experienced by the client. If people with cancer and in palliative care are unable to support their own weight, shearing and sliding should be avoided or kept to a minimum in order to avoid exacerbating pressure sores. Treatment of a person with spinal cord compression will aim to achieve optimum functional independence, although this might only progress as far as being hoisted.

A lifting pole or monkey pole can enable clients to pull themselves up in bed but can also create stress on the shoulders and back, so it is important to consider contraindications. A rope ladder may help clients to pull themselves up but often, by the time they are having difficulties with this sort of movement, they may be too weak to use this.

A mattress variator is expensive but can enable clients to adjust their position in bed. This not only gives the client some independence but it helps the nursing staff or carers avoid the need to assist in lifting the client up the bed or helping him or her sit up. Similarly a leg-lifter attached to the edge of the bed enables the client to transfer in and out of bed independently if he or she finds lifting legs in and out is a problem but care must be taken if the client has leg oedema.

A simpler form of leg-lifter consists of 90 cm of reinforced webbing strap with a loop at one end which is hooked over the instep. The client can then lift the leg up. This is kinder to the leg than hooking the foot with an upside-down walking stick.

A back-rest can support the client comfortably and help him or her sit up in bed – lying down is often a problem for patients with dyspnoea.

Transfer, or sliding, boards can be used to bridge the gap between two surfaces, such as bed and wheelchair, but does involve an element of shearing so the occupational therapist has to be aware of potential hazards. The arm of the wheelchair needs to be removable and 'banana-shaped' transfer boards enable safe and easy transfers. The turning-disc/turntable also assists the carer to transfer the client by rotating, but great care is required in assessing the appropriate-ness of this as the carer needs to have complete control in blocking the client's knees when transferring.

Hoists have been far more widely used in the past few years since lifting and handling regulations were introduced. The decision to provide this equipment depends on whether nursing or home-care staff are to use it in a trained and confident manner or whether members of the family will be the principal users.

When using a hoist, the client should be comfortably supported in the sling. Head support should be provided if necessary. Figure 3.3 illustrates this.

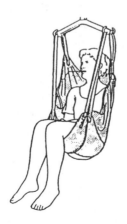

Figure 3.3: A hoist

The ward-based models are likely to be much larger than domestic ones. When a domestic hoist is provided in the client's home, the occupational therapist should assess whether there should also be a nursing bed as the hoist might not fit under a standard bed. In selecting a hoist, there are six main points to be considered:

- the client;
- the carer;
- the task for which the hoist is intended;
- the environment;
- the equipment itself;
- the cost involved.

Alternative transfer techniques should be explored before a hoist is issued as it is a large item of equipment to place in someone's home. It has to be acceptable to the client and carers and there needs to be sufficient room for storing it and manoeuvring it. The operator needs to be properly trained in managing the lifting mechanism and slings.

Overlay mattresses for pressure relief increase the overall height of a bed and this can influence the choice of a hospital bed.

On/off armchair

Electrically operated reclining/riser chairs are extremely expensive and may be seen as a luxury. Some clients will be unable to lie in bed and will only be able to position themselves comfortably in a recliner chair. This equipment could prove cost-effective when clients are discharged from hospital to their homes as it could enable them to position themselves and transfer without assistance.

Equipment for Disabled People (1992) points out some safety factors with these chairs:

- The occupational therapist should not try to raise or alter the height of a recliner chair as this affects the mechanism.
- Self-riser chairs are not suitable for clients with physical dysfunctions such as poor head and trunk control or an inability to lean forward.
- Chairs fitted with manual raising mechanisms which are controlled by the user's body weight must be set up accurately and should not be used if balance is affected.
- The arm-rests must rise with the chair for stability or extend forward to provide a secure lever.

- These chairs are heavy and castors must be fitted for ease of moving, although the chair must be prevented from rolling during transfers.

A well-upholstered armchair with good lumbar and head support is needed for comfort and ease of transfers. The height of the back and arm-rests, the seat depth and the angle of the back are all issues to consider. Specially designed equipment can be used to raise the armchair. Adding pillows or cushions may help if the problem is minor but the client is just as likely to sink back into the cushions and not gain any benefit.

On/off WC

If the WC is accessible, a simple removable raised toilet seat and surround can be added, or a rail- or floor-fixed frame depending on the individual's needs. If hand co-ordination for cleaning oneself is a problem, further assessment is required, for example for a portable bidet. This is filled with warm water, placed in the toilet bowl and the client sits over it to wash. After use, it is tipped backwards so the water pours into the toilet. These are particularly useful for clients with vaginal disease, anal/rectal tumours and offensive discharge.

Should problems arise with catheter or stoma bags, referral is needed to the specialist nurse who can arrange for advice and community support.

Some clients in oncology and palliative care are emaciated and benefit from a padded toilet-seat cover. If they are weak and find transfers an effort, wall-fixed grabrails are firm and safe to use, although the raised seat may cause difficulties in positioning the body when having a bowel motion so the feet may be put on a small step to raise the knees and removed after use, before transferring off the seat.

In/out bath or shower

Depending on the severity of the client's disability, the client's bathroom may need some alteration. This could vary from the provision of simple aids to major adaptations.

Although bathing aids may not be available from social services, or may not be seen by them as a high priority, the occupational therapist should look into the need for such aids in certain cases. If the client has recently undergone surgery or has lymphorrhea, for example, his or her quality of life will be greatly improved if he or she is able to wash thoroughly over the bath.

Bathing aids should preferably be padded as the client is very likely to be emaciated. This not only provides greater comfort in bathing but also prevents injury to an area which is vulnerable to shearing and pressure sores.

The occupational therapist will need to explain the client's needs carefully when referring the matter to social services. The diagnosis might not meet their criteria but associated symptoms and problems might do so.

In palliative care, bath-seats may be less useful as a great deal of arm strength is needed to push oneself up from the seat. If clients are able to achieve that movement, they may choose to actually get down into the bath. Bathing aids should be fully assessed either using a dry or wet trial run in order to decide on the correct combination of equipment. Ideally, a padded hydraulic bath lift can give the client access to a comfortable bath although the rest of the family might find it cumbersome and might not wish to use it. It can be too heavy to lift in and out.

Installation of a lifting device may be more cost-effective than fitting a special bath or shower, although if it necessitates the user sitting with flexed hips and straight knees a standard bathboard or seat may be more useful.

If too much effort is needed when transferring down into the bath, a showerboard over the bath with a flexible hose shower might be used. Individual shower trays usually involve stepping over a ledge, so safety needs to be checked and a hand rail and seat will be needed. It is important that a thermostatically controlled shower system is used to avoid temperature fluctuations and accidental scalding, especially for individuals with impaired sensation.

The form in Appendix 3 can be used to obtain furniture measurements. This is particularly helpful if the assessment in the occupational therapy department has identified the most appropriate item of equipment and all that is needed is the exact measurement – for example, of the bathboard.

Personal and domestic activities of daily living (ADL)

Equipment to aid daily living is essential for clients with limited mobility for whom self-care has become difficult. The energy expended in self-care might push such clients to the limit of their ability to tolerate exercise and the occupational therapist and the client have to establish their priorities and need for carers to assist them.

Toileting equipment has already been discussed. With oncology and palliative care clients it is essential that advice regarding constipation and continence is provided by the multidisciplinary team.

Special attention needs to be paid to skin and dental care, particularly if the client is undergoing treatment. It is important to be aware of the risk of infection. Hygiene must be emphasized and help should be provided if peripheral weakness causes dysfunction.

Hair and nail care can be facilitated using lightweight, long-handled combs and brushes with angled heads or large grips. The appliance officer may be necessary to advise on wigs.

Depending on the disability in question, daily domestic activities can be facilitated using a varied range of equipment from perching stools, tap-turners, helping-hands, kettle/teapot tippers, jar/bottle openers, buttering boards, peelers, knives, cutlery and crockery. It might, however, be the case that the client really needs the help of another person due to fatigue and inability to cope; in this case no item of equipment will be of use.

Standard occupational therapy assessments of washing, dressing and domestic activities of daily living can be carried out on the ward, at the occupational therapy department or in the client's home.

The Structured Observational Test of Function (SOTOF) uses occupational therapy skills to identify problem areas simply and quickly. Although it does not profess to meet everyone's needs, it can be an extremely useful tool for assessing and evaluating clients' progress. The Barthel index can be useful as an indicator but it is not sufficiently sensitive to give a clear picture of performance. The index is often found to give a client a high score when occupational therapists can quickly identify that the same client is not managing at all. Categorizing clients using number scores is a useful way of note-keeping and gaining an idea of the client's abilities but it does not provide the detailed information that is necessary for rehabilitation and functional independence.

There is no one assessment that meets everyone's needs so occupational therapists should remember to qualify the results of any of their assessment techniques with their professional comments about the individual.

The likelihood of improvement in a client's illness is influenced by the stage that the disease has reached. If the client shows little chance of functional improvement, the occupational therapist needs to refer the matter for assessment for the appropriate level of home care for support. Additional help may be required to support the client and family. This help depends on what resources are available locally and includes district nursing, hospice-at-home and voluntary services. If an attendance allowance has been granted, these funds can contribute towards extra assistance, so each individual case needs to be assessed as it arises. In the United Kingdom, referral should be made to social services for an attendance allowance under the special rules that enable the client to obtain funding urgently.

Cognition

The reason for cognitive assessment in occupational therapy is to establish how cognition affects functional independence, both physically and mentally. It is a fascinating area of work. There are a variety of cognitive (and perceptual) assessments that occupational therapists can use and, as with personal and domestic activities of daily living (ADL) assessment, different services will use their own. If, however, the client has a cognitive dysfunction that is affecting his or her lifestyle beyond functional independence, referral to a clinical psychologist may be necessary for assessment and advice.

The occupational therapy process establishes how a client's behaviour differs from what is accepted as 'normal'. It identifies the dysfunction, and formulates the treatment programme.

Normal cognition enables individuals to:

- isolate relevant features of a task;
- formulate a plan;
- break a task down into steps;
- perform actions/behaviour in the correct sequence;
- modify the response when appropriate.

High-level functions can be affected by primary or metastatic brain lesions and also by side effects of treatment. If cognitive impairment is reversible (as in the case of hypercalcaemia) the occupational therapist needs to assess and identify the dysfunction and refer the condition for appropriate treatment.

If there is cerebral metastasis or other neurological damage, the medical team needs to establish the extent of the damage and the likelihood and time span of deterioration. There may be hemiparesis or hemiplegia accompanying this, which may resolve with radiotherapy and chemotherapy. Occupational therapy intervention should aim for maximum recovery. If recovery is poor, compensation and adaptation techniques need to be employed. Similarly, as perceptual difficulties are identified, they need to be addressed using the same problem-solving approach.

Cognitive skills of concern to the occupational therapist will be:

- attention;
- memory – short-term memory being the most relevant in functional independence;
- planning and problem-solving.

Grieve (1993) states that '[a]ttention is closely linked to perception in all human occupation.' She distinguishes between:

- focused attention: the ability to process one input and ignore others;
- attention capacity: the ability to shift attention from one task to another and to do two things at the same time;
- automatic and controlled processing. Automatic processes are fast, do not require attention and are difficult to modify; controlled ones are slow and demand attention but are flexible when circumstances change.

Shifts of attention are important for flexibility in behaviour and action. Attention is closely linked to memory and severe memory impairment presents as the inability to learn and retain new information. This can cause difficulties in planning, sequencing and carrying out activities. In extreme cases, the client forgets what he or she is doing.

Aide-mémoires (such as a diary, a calendar and reminders) pinned up around the house can help, and repeated practice in daily living tasks can assist. By the time the dysfunction becomes particularly severe, the solution is one-to-one supervision.

No one standardized battery of cognitive assessments has proved to cover all needs. Tests are very tiring for the client and time-consuming for the occupational therapist. Our experience is that dysfunction is usually identified during functional assessments if it is significant.

At the risk of seeming defeatist, depending on the reason for cognitive dysfunction, the client may be unlikely to improve significantly once the problem becomes severe. So, compensation and coping mechanisms are the most appropriate approach. This requires establishing with the carer and client how they can construct their daily routine, what help is required, and how to manage with the dysfunction.

Villemoes (1995) wrote of her work with cognitive disorders:

> At the end of rehabilitation the occupational therapy intervention is directed towards:

- stabilisation of the relearned functions and skills,
- compensation of dysfunctions,
- supporting the patient in making realistic plans for the future,
- supporting the patient and the relatives to cope with the altered person,
- supporting integration of the relearned functions, skills and the compensation technique in the patient's daily life in relation to ADL, work, leisure and social life.

These comments referred specifically to stroke and other brain-damaged clients, but they relate well to the area of cognitive impairment in oncology and palliative care.

Occupational therapy in upper-limb dysfunction

Assessment of upper-limb dysfunction in oncology and palliative care patients is similar to such assessment in other fields including rheumatoid and osteoarthritis, as can be seen in Appendix 4.

Prognosis depends entirely on the individual's diagnosis, surgical intervention and radiotherapy. Once a dysfunction has been identified, the occupational therapist chooses the appropriate method of intervention. A splint may be the treatment of choice and, as with all splints, it needs to be specifically designed to keep the affected joint immobile whilst giving support and freedom of movement to other areas.

Dysfunction may be due to:

- side effects of chemotherapy;
- side effects of radiotherapy;
- direct effects of primary tumour;
- direct effects of metastases;
- effects of surgery;
- spinal cord compression
- lymphoedema.

Cook and Burkhardt (1994) describe how chemotherapy causes peripheral neuropathy by demyelinization of the nerve fibres and how it affects large fibre sensory nerves. The resulting symptoms are muscle cramps and/or 'electric shocks' suggesting damage to the posterior column or spinal dorsal nerve column. Partial denervation may result in 'parasthesias, hyperasthesias, complaints of clumsiness when attempting to sustain a grip and impairment or loss of proprioception' (Holden and Felde, 1987).

Difficulties with functional tasks are often reported as well as weakness and atrophy of intrinsic and extrinsic muscle groups, a loss of integrity of the palmar arches and a decreased range of motion of the joints. There is also an increased risk of injury due to sensory changes. Once the drugs are metabolized, and once treatment finishes, the symptoms usually resolve. It is important that the occupational therapist assists the client to maintain a range of motion and optimum independence until this occurs as it is difficult to predict the level of return of sensation and function.

Splinting can help in this area as might an 'activities of daily living' treatment programme based on a problem-solving approach, i.e. washing, dressing and feeding practice to use the hand and arm in such a way as to optimize their functioning. This will not only facilitate independence but will help clients to accept a change in their body image, and a change in their functional status and will prevent feelings of loss and despair often associated with an inability to perform valued activities.

Radiation-induced brachial plexus impairment is discussed in Chapter 4. The treatment goals are mainly palliative, preventative and supportive:

> [C]linical management often includes range of motion of the entire limb, patient education on safety and protection of the desensitized hand, positioning of the upper extremity with slings for comfort or protection, oedema control techniques, static and dynamic splinting of the hand and provision of assistive devices and instruction in compensatory techniques for ADLs. (Cook and Burkhardt, 1994.)

Primary tumours involved in upper-limb dysfunction may include neurological tumours, tumours of the brain or spinal cord, and myelomas. Brain tumours affecting hand function present in hemiparesis or hemiplegia.

Treatments such as radiotherapy are planned to bring about the return of function. As the condition is likely to deteriorate initially due to inflammation in the early stages of radiotherapy, the treatment plan's flexibility will help the client cope. As the radiotherapy takes effect, hand function should improve, although the actual prognosis of the disease may require the occupational therapist to plan ahead in the case of likely deterioration.

Myeloma may cause bone marrow pathology resulting in spinal cord compression, carpal tunnel syndrome and peripheral neuropathy. Bone tenderness and pathological fractures may also occur and, again, the occupational therapy intervention involves gentle maintenance of function and adaptation to decreased abilities. Similarly, metastatic disease, for example from breast or lung primary tumours, can affect the nervous system, the spinal cord,

nerve roots or peripheral nerve fibres and the occupational therapist's aims are focused towards adaptation rather than returning to
full function.

Clients experiencing upper-limb dysfunction with a diagnosis of
cancer may continue to deteriorate functionally. This is discussed
further in Chapter 4. Each client needs to be assessed on an individual basis and discussion may be necessary with the surgeon or radiol-
ogist. Follow-up appointments and ongoing evaluation are necessary
to ensure adequate future planning is provided should the condition
worsen.

Clothing and dressing

Difficulties relating to clothing do not simply stop at the physical act
of getting dressed or undressed. Clothing is a statement by the
wearer about their culture, mood and freedom of choice. Body
image needs to be addressed in many cases when considering the
issue of clothing.

Children, adolescents and adults will all have their own preferences and an individual with a disability may feel particularly strongly
about his or her body image. If clients are unable to go shopping, they
should be involved in consultation about their wardrobe.

Mass production of clothing makes it affordable and specialized
garments are likely to be more expensive. The occupational therapist should analyse the specific difficulties the client has in negotiating clothing and should establish the most appropriate solution.

Adaptations and advice regarding clothing and dressing for
clients in oncology and palliative care depend on the individual's
difficulties. These may include:

* poor fine finger co-ordination (a particular problem where fasten-
  ings are concerned);
* weakness, shortness of breath and fatigue;
* limited mobility, inability to stand and inability to adjust clothing;
* problems with pressure sores;
* open wounds and leaking requiring clothing to be protected;
* incontinence;
* lymphoedema;
* hemiplegia or paraplegia.

If the client's skin is sensitive due to radiotherapy or neuropathy, he
or she needs to be aware of fabrics and how they affect body temperature. Particular attention needs to be given to the use of natural

fibres and which detergents are used. There may be a particular area of the body that has the potential to rub and care must be taken to avoid this.

With regard to incontinence:

> Careful planning of one's wardrobe brings increased independence and confidence so that incontinence becomes less frequent. Inability to manage clothing – manipulating trouser fastenings, pulling pants up and down – can be overcome by wearing specially adapted or designed clothes.
>
> In general, clothes which do not have to be removed over the head are the most convenient. Seams and fastenings should be kept to a minimum as they are likely to become soiled and are harder to get completely clean. Large amounts of clothing are needed when there is severe incontinence. (Equipment for Disabled People, 1989.)

In order to prevent catheter tubing catching in clothing, it can be arranged not to snag. This can be accomplished, for example, by using split-back nightwear, split-back dresses or wrap-around clothing. Leg bags enable ease of emptying and better drainage.

Advice should be sought from a specialist stoma nurse as to whether clients with a stoma can continue to wear ordinary clothes. Positioning and care of the bag can be arranged so that it is not visible and one need not necessarily change one's dress habits.

Clients with a mastectomy may choose to wear a prosthesis or have reconstructive surgery. Underwear and swimwear is readily available for prosthetic users and appliance officers and specialist breast-care nurses can advise on techniques and suppliers for managing this.

Loose-fitting clothing is often the most comfortable solution for clothing problems as it facilitates easier dressing and undressing. It need not necessarily comprise baggy jogging suits. Long jumpers are easily available and they can cover muscle bulk loss or take emphasis away from amputation. Stretchable lycra clothing is easy to remove and put on.

Footwear can be difficult, particularly if feet and legs are oedematous. Specialist suppliers manufacture wide, easily removable flat shoes. Ordinary shoe shops can provide smart flat shoes although these might not be sufficiently large to accommodate the client.

Clients' clothing problems need to be assessed and addressed as they occur. Dressing aids and techniques – for example, one-handed dressing – are well known to occupational therapists and are well documented.

Body image involves more than clothing. For this reason it may be necessary to provide advice on hair, make-up and shaving as well as counselling from a specialist.

Summary

Assessment and treatment are continuous and ongoing processes. It is important to:

- set realistic goals with the client and carer;
- draw from clinical experience and use core occupational therapy skills;
- enable the client and carer to achieve optimum functional independence.

It is equally important to recognize:

- when the client and carer have achieved their goals;
- when the client deteriorates.

More specific intervention is discussed in Chapter 4.

Action points

1. Identify and document legislation specific to social services guidelines regarding provision of services for oncology and palliative care clients in your local area. How would you approach such service providers to improve the urgency of services?
2. Establish which items of equipment are readily available for acute and long-term disabilities. Which items take longer to provide? Which requests for items need to go before a panel of assessors for consideration due to expense? How could this be overcome?
3. Describe the processes and procedures required in the analysis of your clients' problems. Outline the treatment programmes and interventions required.
4. What unique aspects need to be considered in planning treatment for a client in an oncology and palliative care setting as compared to one in an acute surgical unit?

References

College of Occupational Therapists (1995) Manual Handling Operations Regulations 1992 and their Application Within Occupational Therapy. London: College of Occupational Therapists.

Cook A, Burkhardt A (1994) The effect of cancer diagnosis and treatment on hand function. American Journal of Occupational Therapy 48(9): 836–9.

Equipment for Disabled People (1989) Clothing and Dressing. Oxford: The Disability Information Trust.

Equipment for Disabled People (1992) Furniture. Oxford: The Disability Information Trust.

Equipment for Disabled People (1995) Home Management and Housing. Oxford: The Disability Information Trust.

Equipment for Disabled People (1990) Personal Care. Oxford: The Disability Information Trust.

Grieve J (1993) Neuropsychology for occupational therapists. Oxford: Blackwell Science.

Hagopian G (1993) Cognitive strategies used in adapting to a cancer diagnosis. Oncology Nursing Forum 20(5): 759–63.

Hens M (1989) Functional evaluation. In Dittmar S (Ed) Rehabilitation Nursing Process and Application. St Louis: CV Mosby, p. 487.

Holden S, Felde G (1987) Nursing care of patients experiencing cisplatin-related peripheral neuropathy. Oncology Nursing Forum 14(1): 13–19.

Merton Social Services (1994) Practice Note on Registration as a Disabled Person. London: Merton Social Services.

Pedretti L, Zolton B (1990) Occupational Therapy, Practice Skills for Physical Dysfunction. St Louis: CV Mosby.

Villemoes Sorenson L (1995) The Occupational Therapy intervention of patients with cognitive disorders in Denmark. WFOT Bulletin 32: 33–5.

Watson P (1992) Cancer rehabilitation – an overview. Seminars in Oncology Nursing 8(3): 169.

World Health Organization (1980) International Classification of Impairments, Disabilities and Handicaps. WHO: Geneva.

Further reading

Baxandall S, Reddy P (1993) The Courage To Care. Melbourne: David Lovell Publishing.

Eggers O (1983) Occupational Therapy in the Treatment of Adult Hemiplegia. London: Heinemann.

Mill D, Fraser C (1989) Therapeutic Activities for the Upper Limb. Oxford: Winslow Press.

Payne R (1995) Relaxation Techniques. Edinburgh: Churchill Livingstone.

Reed K (1991) Quick Reference to Occupational Therapy. Aspen, Maryland: Gaithersbury.

Turner A (1990) The Practice of Occupational Therapy. Edinburgh: Churchill Livingstone.

Chapter 4
Occupational Therapy in Specific Symptom Control and Dysfunction

Jill Cooper

This chapter discusses how occupational therapy intervention addresses symptom control. It looks at problem-solving, feeding, the assessment and prescription of wheelchairs, the healing of wounds and pressure sores, radiation-induced brachial plexopathy, spinal-cord compression and dyspnoea. It also explores the limitations of occupational therapy, particularly with regard to pain control, nausea and vomiting.

Occupational therapists make a valuable contribution in alleviating certain symptoms. Their intervention is symptom-led rather than disease- or diagnosis-led and they deal with each functional problem as it presents itself. They also try to anticipate problems so that they are prepared for them.

Dunlop (1989) listed the 12 common symptoms treated in palliative care as:

weakness 82%	swollen legs 46%
dry mouth 68%	nausea 42%
anorexia 58%	constipation 36%
depression 52%	vomiting 32%
pain 46%	confusion 30%
insomnia 46%	dyspnoea 30%

Problem-solving

Occupational therapy intervention takes a 'problem-solving' approach to symptom control. Problem-solving forms the basis for analysing the client's needs and enabling the client to cope with dysfunction. Illness creates physical, psychological, emotional, social and financial problems. Even though a client's situation can appear overwhelming, the occupational therapist will find it helpful to identify specific problems and to try to resolve them.

In all occupational therapy treatment plans, the first step is to establish rapport and to set baseline aims and objectives. The problem-solving strategy can then be set out. In anxiety management, for example, a strategy might involve the following:

• trying to identify the underlying difficulty;
• establishing and discussing the particular event that might contribute to the initiation of the problem;
• setting achievable aims to deal with that event by breaking the problem down into stages;
• discussing techniques and methods to cope with these stages;
• discussion of what the outcome might be if the problem-solving strategy succeeds and of what to do next;
• making it clear that the strategy might not always succeed but that it is necessary to persevere.

This would enable the patient to apply techniques themselves and cope with anxiety-provoking situations.

Sheila Cassidy (1991) offers the following advice:

• Make sure that you are quite clear about the patient's history at the outset. Read the notes and be sure of the facts.
• See the patient alone and in privacy, not with relatives or behind curtains.
• Introduce yourself.
• Explain that you know about the case.
• Take notes thoroughly when the client gives you his or her story. It can be frustrating for the patient to tell the story for the ninth time but you do need to get the facts down.
• Discover what the patient wants to know.
• Explain about the illness and be honest.
• Establish the prognosis in order to establish the timescale within which you are working.
• Hold a closing interview, summing up and making a plan for the next stage of treatment.

Equipment

When providing equipment the occupational therapist should consider:

- whether equipment needs to be adjusted regularly and how safely this can be done;
- comfort;
- acceptance of equipment;
- safety;
- durability and quality;
- cleaning;
- transportation and storage;
- repairs and spares;
- price and availability of resources;
- how the equipment is to be evaluated.

The occupational therapist should remember that equipment is not the answer to everything.

Pain control

Seventy per cent of clients experience pain and it is more commonly seen in cancers of the pancreas and oesaphagus (30–90%) than others (for example, less than 50% of lymphoma sufferers report pain). Kaye (1994) explains that bone pain accounts for 40% of cancer pain. Bone pain tends to be exacerbated by movement. It is localized and sensitive to pressure and percussion. The treatment of choice is radiotherapy and relief often occurs within days.

Turk and Fernandez (1991) write that:

> The influence of the situation in which the pain occurs on the perceived level of pain is particulary important in cancer patients because of the fear and anxiety often evoked by the diagnosis.

Although occupational therapists do work on pain control with chronic pain syndromes, clients in the oncology and palliative care setting are in a different situation. Their medication has to be correctly supervised by palliative care specialists in order to achieve optimum pain control or relief. Symptom control in palliative care does not have the same behavioural and cognitive element as chronic pain control does.

A publication entitled *Guidelines for Managing Cancer Pain in Adults* by the National Council for Hospice and Specialist Palliative Care Services (1994) explains that pain is one of the most common, and still one of the most feared, symptoms of cancer. Many patients have more than one pain and not all pain is caused by cancer (for example there will also be pain caused by surgery and post-herpetic neuralgia).

The problem of pain control is complicated by the fact that pain thresholds and tolerance vary between individuals. Table 4.1 outlines some of the more common types of pain experienced by cancer sufferers. Cancer pain is usually divided into the following categories: visceral, soft tissue, bone, nerve and secondary visceral spasm (in the gut, bladder and rectum).

Breakthrough pain may occur before the next regular dose of analgesia is due. *Incident pain* occurs with movement, when a vulnerable part of the body has to bear weight, and when a dressing is being changed.

Pharmacological management

Mild pain:

- Paracetomol
- NSAID

Moderate pain:

- Weak opioids used in combination with the simple analgesics used to treat mild pain.
- Dextropropoxyphene

or

- Codeine/dihydrocodeine

Severe pain:

- Strong opioids, oral morphine.

Medical and nursing staff adjust morphine as appropriate depending on the individual's needs. Side effects of pain control include nausea and vomiting, constipation, drowsiness and urinary retention. Respiratory depression is very rare.

Tolerance and dependence may occur, but physical dependence is not to be confused with addiction. Cancer patients who require opioids for pain do not manifest evidence of psychological dependence and fear of causing addiction cannot be used as a reason to withhold opioids from cancer pain patients.

Alternative strong opioids, adjuvant (co-analgesics), radiotherapy, neural blockade and surgery may also play a role in pain relief.

Table 4.1: Common pain problems in cancer patients
(From Guidelines for Managing Cancer Pain in Adults, National Council for Hospice and Specialist Palliative Care Service)

	Examples	Character	Location	Clinical findings
Superficial pain	Pressure areas Subcutaneous metastases	Sharp	Well-localized	Inflammation Ulceration Tenderness
Deep somatic pain	Bone metastases	Dull, aching Pain on weight-bearing or movement	Relatively localized	Decreased range of motion
Visceral pain	Liver metastases Bowel obstruction	Dull, aching Colic	Relatively localized	Tender organomegaly
Nerve (neuropathic) pain	Brachial plexopathy (e.g. in breast cancer) Lumbosacral plexopathy (e.g. rectal cancer, cervical cancer) Cranial nerve involvement (e.g. head and neck cancer)	Burning, shooting, stabbing, sometimes aching	Referred to distribution of damaged nerve/s	Altered sensation Allodynia i.e. non-painful stimuli, such as light touch, cause pain Motor weakness Altered reflexes

Pharmacological pain control takes place at several levels (Kaye, 1994). These are:

- nerve endings;
- peripheral nerves;
- the dorsal horn;
- the spino-thalamic tract;
- the midbrain;
- the cortex.

Other interventions for clients with pain

Anxiety- and stress-management techniques will not directly help control pain but they can help patients cope with it. Occupational therapy needs to concentrate on the physical and psychological approaches to pain. Turk and Fernandez (1991) write that:

> Pain is a multidimensional experience with sensory as well as cognitive and affective components affected by environmental contingencies.

Each component needs to be addressed by a multifaceted approach. It is important to acknowledge that the association between pain and psychological distress in cancer patients may be one of reciprocal causality. Pain is likely to cause distress and psychological distress can increase the patient's perception of pain.

Spiegel and Bloom (1983) found that mood disturbance and the meaning of pain to a patient was related to the patient's reported pain intensity in a sample of 86 females with metastatic breast cancer. They reported that greater mood disturbance and the belief that pain signalled a worsening of their disease were significantly correlated with reported pain intensity.

In anxiety and stress management sessions, the client may derive benefit from just being allowed to talk about pain (or other problems) – to identify what initiates it, how it manifests itself, what to do about it and how to reduce anxiety. Lloyd and Coggles (1988) state that

> [i]t is important to understand the significance of the pain experienced by the individual and provide assistance in the areas of life that are viewed as being important to them. . . . Pain control is a necessity for living so that the individual can continue to carry out, to the extent that he is able, his chosen life tasks and roles in the time that is left.

Occupational therapy involves assessing what is needed for the patient's comfort and arranging for mattress variators, wheelchairs, equipment for seating and positioning, and pressure relief (especially where there are pressure sores). It can also involve providing advice on implementing care.

Nausea and vomiting

Black and Morrow (1991) write that:

> Nausea and vomiting are among the most prevalent, persistent and undesirable side effects of cancer chemotherapy treatment.

Kaye (1994) reports that the incidence of nausea and vomiting is 50% of clients with advanced cancer and 30% on admission to hospice. Medical intervention depends on the causes. These might include:

- drugs
- anxiety
- brain metastases
- oral thrush
- gastric irritation
- squashed stomach syndrome
- gastric outflow obstruction
- constipation
- cough

Nausea and vomiting are distressing and can lead to anorexia, dehydration, an upset in metabolic balance and even depression. They can manifest themselves before or after chemotherapy. Neither responds well to antiemetics and antiemetics themselves can produce side effects of anxiety.

Studies have shown positive results from progressive muscular relaxation training. This enables the patient to take some control and relax (Payne, 1995). It can also reduce the side effects both during and after a course of cancer chemotherapy.

The occupational therapist should find the most suitable method to manage anxiety for the client. This should enable the client to recognize the onset of a nauseous episode, practise the relaxation technique and avoid an episode of anxiety which could result in nausea and vomiting. It is equally important in this setting to recognize one's own limitations and to know when to refer the matter to a clinical psychologist.

The occupational therapist contemplating the use of anxiety- and stress-management techniques must be aware of contraindications.

If a client is depressed rather than anxious, he or she should be referred for psychiatric help. Be cautious in selecting clients for individual or group relaxation sessions. Group dynamics have an effect on the outcome of such techniques. Criteria should be established for selecting clients for inclusion in such groups.

Payne (1995) writes that:

> Imagery and visualization methods are not suitable for people suffering from severe mental disorders. Imagery is particularly inadvisable for people who have difficulty in separating fantasy from reality and for those who experience hallucinations.

Feeding problems

Occupational therapists can help clients with their feeding. Feeding is such a basic aspect of daily living that it is very important that any problems with this activity are understood.

Difficulties in feeding oneself independently may take the form of problems with hand–eye co-ordination or with swallowing. Clients with cancer and in palliative care may also experience nausea, may lack appetite and may find that their sense of taste has altered because of disease or treatment. All these problems need to be addressed by the dietitian.

Weight loss may be caused by ill-fitting teeth, oral infections and ulcers, as well as changes in taste.

Physical feeding problems requiring advice and assessment by the occupational therapist are likely to manifest themselves in the client being unable to actually get food to the mouth. This should be analysed and tackled using a variety of techniques and equipment, including adapted cutlery, crockery and non-slip mats. The occupational therapist should also be aware of problems with the actual supply of food, such as problems in preparing meals, or in carrying food from the kitchen to the dining area. Again, the difficulty needs to be analysed and appropriate techniques and equipment (such as trolleys) should be considered.

Feeding problems can give rise to psychological difficulties. Energy intake (calorie intake) and mood are directly related so reduction in food intake can cause negative changes in mood. Clients who are unable to eat well may feel guilty because they are not eating and this in turn upsets their carers. Sometimes it can be helpful to distract the client's attention away from food – for example, by giving the client a foot-rub so that something useful and pleasant is being offered.

Loss of appetite occurs in approximately 70% of clients. Possible causes include drugs, anxiety or depression, constipation, nausea, oral thrush and mouth ulcers. The gut is a muscle and needs to work to stay in good functional order. If one eats less, the capacity to eat reduces.

It is important to consider the following points when assessing the needs of clients with a poor appetite:

- It might be advisable for the client to have small amounts of food as large portions on a plate can be extremely offputting.
- The frequency of these small portions can be increased.
- The client should eat food that does not require too much effort. Bread and meat, for example, are difficult to chew. This does not mean clients should have steamed fish and soft boiled eggs, nor do they have to be fed Guinness and beef sandwiches! Puddings, particularly ready-made ones, are ideal: they are small, ready whenever they are wanted and do not give rise to feelings of guilt because no one goes to a great effort to provide a pudding, so if it is not eaten it does not matter.
- Clients should eat what they want whenever they want. There is no reason why they should keep to the pattern of breakfast, lunch and evening meal.
- Appetite often reduces later in the day so it might be advisable to try the largest meal earlier.

If the client has cravings, indulge them. Encourage the intake of high-energy food (high-calorie food). Energy is more important than protein in these circumstances. Fat is the richest source of calories and when a client's appetite is very small (as is often the case whilst undergoing chemotherapy) the client needs the maximum amount of energy in the smallest amount of food. Some clients will express concern about raising their cholesterol levels. They should be reassured that their need for additional energy is of far greater importance than any potential long-term consequences from an increased cholesterol level. (Long-term consequences will sadly not be an issue for many of these clients.)

Alcohol is high in energy and should be allowed unless specifically forbidden by the doctor. It is also an appetite stimulant with a direct effect on the gut and it reduces the effects of anxiety, making eating easier. Furthermore, it is customary to take wine or beer with food, so alcohol helps the client to maintain some elements of a 'normal' lifestyle.

Functional independence in feeding

It is important to promote independence in feeding for the following reasons:

- It helps clients' feelings of morale and dignity if they can feed themselves.
- Feeding is the one of earliest skills learned and one of the last skills to be lost. Loss of this skill emphasizes a person's dependence.
- It can be very frustrating to be fed by someone else as people all have individual differences and habits in their eating.
- Encouraging the development of feeding skills motivates clients to improve other areas of functional independence.
- Food and meal times are very much a social activity.
- Feeding a sick person is extremely time-consuming for the carer.

There are, of course, always cases where independent eating is neither feasible nor appropriate. Clients with a gross tremor of the head and/or hand, or who become tired extremely quickly on exertion, may prefer to be fed and conserve their energies for other activities.

When feeding someone it is necessary to establish the order in which that person likes to eat food, the preferred size of the mouth-fuls and the preferred speed of eating.

An inability to feed independently might arise if certain skills and attributes are lacking. These include:

- eyesight;
- an adequate range of movement;
- muscle strength in the arms/hands;
- hand function;
- head control;
- posture;
- recognition of food/utensils/body parts;
- sensation (hot/cold/stereognosis);
- decision making;
- ability to plan, execute and sequence movements;
- concentration;
- memory;
- orientation;
- motivation;
- comprehension;
- judgement;
- mood;
- level of consciousness.

Environmental and social factors are important in clients' ability to feed themselves. They include:

- access to the dining area;
- access to the table;
- the height of the table and chair;
- the type of chair provided;
- light, warmth, comfort;
- the atmosphere – it should be safe, unhurried and sociable;
- the presentation of food.

Religion, culture and family upbringing all have implications for the development of individual feeding habits. The individual's habits, likes and dislikes should be respected so that he or she can maintain a sense of identity. Meal-times should be associated with communication and sharing. Clients should trust their feeders and feel that they have their respect. If the client is dependent and does not enjoy being fed, this can result in refusal to eat, confusion and extreme weakness.

Rejection of food may be due to:

- poor positioning and discomfort;
- dislike;
- poor appetite;
- inability to chew food adequately;
- attention-seeking to express frustration;
- reduced taste and smell perception;
- the texture of the food;
- cultural aspects.

A person who is poorly positioned may feel uncomfortable. This may divert his or her attention from the task and could be hazardous. It may cause difficulties with swallowing. (Specific difficulties with swallowing should be referred to the speech therapist and dietitian as there may be an obstruction.) Poor positioning means that increased effort is required to carry out the necessary movements and that enjoyment is reduced.

When positioning a client, aim for symmetry and a position which allows isolated movements of the head, trunk and limbs. The client should sit erect, with the spine and neck slightly extended. Both buttocks should bear the client's weight. The feet should be firmly on the floor or on the footplates of the wheelchair. Comfort can be improved by choosing the appropriate type of chair and by ensuring that the height of the chair is correct in relation to the table.

The occupational therapist should be aware of any problems concerning:

- posture;
- psychological attitude (this should include an awareness of previous experiences, atmosphere and the attitude of the carer);
- diet (liquids can be harder to swallow than semi-solids);
- the temperature of food: extremes of temperature tend to stimulate coughing or choking.

When finding solutions to problems, the occupational therapist may need to work with the carer to take the following factors into consideration:

- If there is visual impairment, colours and lighting should contrast with the environment and utensils and should make it very clear what food is available. It may be necessary to provide protective garments, non-slip mats, plate guards and crockery with steep sides.
- If the client can eat with one hand only it may be necessary to provide non-slip mats, plate guards, suction egg cups and combined cutlery.
- If the client has a poor ability to grip it may be necessary to provide altered or adapted cutlery with enlarged, lightweight handles and two-handled mugs.
- If the client has poor concentration, or is easily distracted, or is self-conscious, provide a quiet place for eating.
- If there is weakness or fatigue in the arms, provide stabilizing crockery, lightweight cutlery, serrated knives and plate guards.
- If there are problems with co-ordination, ataxia or spasms, provide stabilizing crockery, plastic tableware, equipment to stablize the head and protective garments.
- If there is a tremor, provide equipment to stabilize the wrist, half-fill cups and use deep spoons.
- If there is a limited range of movement, raise the table use long-handled/angled cutlery. Such clients could eat with their forearms on the table, using their elbows as pivots.
- If the client is very slow, provide heated plates and insulated mugs. The client should eat little but often, without hurrying. It is important to ensure that the environment is comfortable.

- If the client has sensory deficits, he or she should avoid very hot foods and fluids. It is possible to use a mirror to train such clients to become aware of the area of altered sensation.

Wheelchair prescription

Equipment for Disabled People (1993) points out that the following factors need to be taken into consideration when prescribing a wheelchair:

- physical measurements of the user and the wheelchair
- the person's disablement and abilities
- social and environmental factors
- cost.

It continues:

A well-chosen wheelchair should maximise the user's mobility, independence, comfort and confidence. The basic requirements are for a stable, adjustable seat, which is easy to use and manoeuvre, both by the disabled person and by any helpers, and which is well-made and of attractive appearance.

The main measurements of the wheelchair are:

- seat width
- seat depth
- seat height
- backrest height
- arm-rest height
- foot-rest length and angle.

Ideally the knee, ankle and elbow joints should be at right angles. For comfort, some users may prefer the backrest to be angled back slightly. The controls and pushing rims should be within reach without having to stretch.

Dysfunction and abilities need to be assessed, particularly:

- the client's ability to propel;
- the method of propulsion (by user or attendant?);
- optimum positioning in the chair;
- weight and balance (this involves considering whether the client has poor balance or whether wheels need setting back due to lower limb amputation);
- modifications;
- method of transfer into and out of the wheelchair;
- the carers' abilities.

Social and environmental factors that should be considered include:

- the width of narrowest doorways and turning spaces;
- manoeuvring spaces;
- passage widths;
- gradient of ramps and inclines;
- the possibility of transporting the wheelchair.

The client in oncology and palliative care may not require a wheelchair permanently and it might be preferable to investigate temporary loan. If the condition is deteriorating, regular evaluation is required to ensure that further help is provided as necessary. This might include the provision of pressure cushions and arm or head supports.

Wounds and pressure sores

Cancer patients often find that there are problems with the healing of wounds. Jones (1978) writes that these are

> all generally related to a decrease in host immunocompetence causing delay in, or problems with, the healing process.

Cancer-related factors include:

- radiotherapy causing tissue hypoxia;
- chemotherapy causing neutropenia;
- malnutrition resulting in lack of sufficient nutrients;
- anaemia causing delay in tissue repair;
- corticosteroid therapy reducing white cell activity;
- disease affecting normal bone marrow stem cells reduces white cell activity and depresses the immune response;
- stress/anxiety increases production of adrenocorticotrophic hormone and corticosteroids.

Basic care of potential pressure areas is essential and is straightforward. Waterlow (1995) writes that

> Pressure sore, bed sore, decubitus ulcer (USA) – from the Latin *decumbare,* to lie down–, are really all misnomers because:
> a. Pressure, though the main factor in causing pressure sores, is not the only one.
> b. People sitting in a chair or wheelchair for long periods, without pressure being relieved, can be at greater risk, as the interface pressures are higher due to the fact that the mass of the body is distributed over a smaller area of tissue.

Occupational therapists have developed specialist skills in the areas of assessment and prescription for wheelchair users. The permanent wheelchair user is likely to have special pressure-care needs and if clients need a special mattress then they need a comparable cushion to complement this when they sit out of bed.

It is not only the wheelchair user in oncology and palliative care who needs specialist attention. When the client sits on an ordinary armchair, the body weight is taken on the ischial tuberosities and tissues. The type of armchair the patient uses therefore also needs to be considered.

Waterlow (1995) explains that:

> if a chair is too low or has a tilted back, the body weight is taken on a smaller area of tissue and the patient has difficulty in standing up. If a chair is too high, all of the body weight is taken on the ischeal tuberosities as the feet and legs are not supporting their own weight. . . . Adjustments should be made to enable the patient to sit with his/her back upright, thighs at an angle of 90 degrees to the body, lower legs at an angle of 90 degrees to the thighs and feet resting comfortably on the ground or a step at an angle of 90 degrees to the lower legs.

The armrests, the back rest, seat depth and footrests must be set up accurately to achieve good posture and decreased pressure.

Pressure sores develop when:

- tissues become distorted due to direct external force on the body;
- the capillaries become occluded as they are squashed between the body's weight and skeleton and the mattress/cushion;
- tissue ischaemia occurs and if not alleviated results in necrosis and then in pressure sores;
- shearing forces cause tissue distortion when a part of the body tries to move but the skin remains still – for example, when the client slips down the bed but the bottom does not actually move on the sheet;
- friction forces occur when there are shearing forces in conjunction with lateral forces – for example, when the draw sheet is dragged from under the client or the heels are dragged along the bed;
- moisture (for example sweating or incontinence) further compromises tissues, adding to the damage to the pressure areas;
- nutrition is decreased, so the body has depleted resources to enable it to heal;
- skin temperature rises.

Clients with blood oxygen levels that drop significantly when sitting appear to be at high risk.

Pressure areas commonly develop over bony prominences (sacrum, heels, ischial tuberosities, back of head, elbows, scapulae, spine, hips, knees and ankles). They can also occur where soft tissues are in contact – for example, under the breasts.

A common risk assessment measurement should be available to the multidisciplinary team. The Waterlow scale is widely recognized and used. The assessment scale provides guidelines on selection and preventative aids and wound classification. It should be borne in mind that the Waterlow scale is devised to look at rehabilitation clients and is not validated for wheelchair users.

Dealey (1995) explains that a

> risk calculator should form only part of the total assessment of the patient . . . However, it is not sufficient for an institution to decide that all patients will be assessed using a risk calculator, education for the user is also required.

The cause of pressure sores is not truly known and risk-assessment scales should only be used in conjunction with a range of other factors and general observations. Transcutaneous gas measurements are now felt to be significant and are being used alongside pressure measurements in some hospitals. This technique is in its early stages.

The following issues are important when assessing risk and planning preventative measures:

- Consideration of the predisposing factors to identify those clients at risk.
- An awareness of skin care, including an awareness of signs of pressure injury.
- Control of incontinence.
- Dietary management.
- Relieving pressure by providing appropriate mattresses and cushions to spread weight distribution.
- Encouraging clients and carers to become aware of the risk of damage to the skin.
- Encouraging clients to change their position frequently.
- Avoiding shearing and friction by using hoists for transfers if the clients are unable to support their own weight.
- Investigating possible ways of decreasing excessive build-ups of moisture.

WOUND CLASSIFICATION
Stirling Pressure Score severity scale (SPSSS)

Stage 0 — No clinical evidence of pressure sore
0.1 — Healed with scarring
0.2 — Tissue damage not assessed as a pressure sore (a) below

Stage 1 — Discoloration of intact skin
1.1 — Non-blanchable erythema with increased local heat
1.2 — Blue/purple/black discoloration — the sore is at least **Stage 1** (a or b)

Stage 2 — Partial thickness skin loss or damage
2.1 — Blister
2.2 — Abrasion
2.3 — Shallow ulcer, no undermining of adjacent tissue
2.4 — Any of these with underlying blue/purple/black discoloration or induration. The sore is at least **Stage 2** (a, b or c+d for **2.3**, +e for **2.4**)

Stage 3 — Full-thickness skin loss involving damage/necrosis of subcutaneous tissue, not extending to underlying bone tendon or joint capsule
3.1 — Crater, without undermining adjacent tissue
3.2 — Crater, with undermining of adjacent tissue
3.3 — Sinus, the full extent of which is uncertain
3.4 — Necrotic tissue masking full extent of damage.
The sore is at least **Stage 3** (b, +/-e, f, g, +h for **3.4**)

Stage 4 — Full-thickness loss with extensive destruction and tissue necrosis extending to underlying bone tendon or capsule
4.1 — Visible exposure of bone tendon or capsule
4.2 — Sinus assessed as extending to same (b+/-e, f, g, h, i)

Guide to types of Dressings/Treatment
a. Semipermeable membrane
b. Hydrocolloid
c. Foam dressing
d. Alginate
e. Hydrogel
f. Alginate rope/ribbon
g. Foam cavity filler
h. Enzymatic debridement
i. Surgical debridement

PREVENTION:
PREVENTATIVE AIDS:

Special Mattress/Bed: 10+ overlays or specialist foam mattresses.
15+ alternating pressure overlays, mattresses and bed systems.
20+ Bed System: Fluidised, bead, low air loss and alternating pressure mattresses.
Note: Preventative aids cover a wide spectrum of specialist features. Efficacy should be judged, if possible, on the basis of independent evidence.

Cushions: No patient should sit in a wheelchair without some form of cushioning. If nothing else is available — use the patient's own pillow.
10+4" Foam cushion.
15+ Specialist cell and/or foam cushion
20+ Cushion capable of adjustment to suit individual patient.

Bed Clothing: Avoid plastic draw sheets, inco pads and tightly tucked in sheets/sheet covers, especially when using Specialist bed and mattress overlay systems.
Use Duvet-plus vapour permeable cover.

NURSING CARE
General: Frequent changes of position, lying/sitting
Use of pillows
Pain Appropriate pain control
Nutrition High protein, vitamins, minerals
Patient Handling: Correct lifting technique – Hoists – Monkey Pole – Transfer Devices
Patient Comfort Aids: Real sheepskins — Bed Cradle
Operating Table
Theatre/A&E Trolley 4" cover plus adequate protection.
Skin Care: General Hygiene, NO rubbing, cover with an appropriate dressing

If treatment is required, first remove pressure

Figure 4.1: The Waterlow scale

The team requires a co-ordinated and standardized approach with nursing procedures, transfers and mobility, nutritional intake and constant use of preventative and therapeutic equipment.

Once an appropriate pressure-relieving cushion is chosen, the occupational therapist needs to establish whether it is for use in the wheelchair or the armchair as this influences who is responsible for its provision. It can be used in either, but if it is to be used primarily in the armchair, this will generally be seen as a nursing need. More complicated queries regarding seating, positioning and pressure care need to be referred to the local wheelchair service, which has expertise to advise on solutions.

Although there are dozens, if not hundreds, of pressure-relieving cushions on the market, a standard selection does assist evaluation and enables the team to familiarize itself with the equipment available.

Clothing can be an important factor in dealing with pressure wounds. Equipment for Disabled People (1989) explains:

> Seams, especially thick double seams, can cause sores if they are in weight bearing areas: under the thighs for those in a wheelchair, under the upper arm for a crutch user, in the small of the back for those lying or sitting for long periods. Abrasive fabrics should be avoided. . . . Warm clothes are needed for comfort and safety but this can conflict with the need for a constant temperature unless they are made in breathable fabrics.

Clothes should allow adequate ventilation in warmer weather and, if skin moisture is a problem, absorbent fabrics can be worn. Encourage regular changes of clothing. Loosely woven non-absorbent, man-made materials such as polyester or polypropylene allow moisture to pass through, leaving the skin dry.

Guidelines for provision of pressure cushions for wheelchairs

Wheelchair pressure-relief cushions should be part of a comprehensive pressure-care management plan for each client. The criteria for provision of such cushions are as follows:

- the client must be registered with the wheelchair service;
- the client should be assessed as 'at risk' on a recognized risk-assessment scale (such as the Norton scale or the Waterlow scale) or should show signs of recent and significant weight loss or poor or deteriorating general health;
- the client must be willing to accept referral to other agencies if appropriate (for example, the community nurse or the regional tissue viability team);

- the client must spend extended periods sitting in a wheelchair, transfer to static seating being inappropriate or not possible;
- the cushion is issued on loan following assessment and at the therapist's discretion;
- the cushion will be selected from the current range provided by the wheelchair service;
- the cushion is provided for use in a wheelchair only;
- the client/carer must agree to carry out any maintenance instructions issued with the cushion and use the cushion as prescribed by the therapist.

The order of priority for the provision of pressure cushions is:

1. Clients with existing pressure sores.
2. Clients assessed at 'high risk' of developing pressure sores.
3. Clients assessed at 'medium risk' of developing pressure sores.
4. Low risk clients.

The assessment and referrals forms can be seen in Appendix 5.

Radiation-induced brachial plexopathy (RIBP)

A relatively high dose of radiation is necessary to sterilize microscopic deposits of breast cancer and survival may be prolonged by high doses of post-operative radiotherapy in selected patients. However, at these levels of radiotherapy there is a relatively steep increase in the risk of complications. The Royal College of Radiologists, together with the Radiation Action Group Exposure (RAGE), have produced guidelines for the management of clients with RIBP, some of which is summarized below.

Clients who have undergone treatment for breast cancer may suffer a range of upper limb problems:

- oedema
- inner-arm sensation changes related to surgery
- more rarely, brachial plexus neuropathy associated with radiation damage.

In a minority of patients, supraclavicular and/or axillary irradiation may cause oedema and fibrous tissue to constrict the brachial plexus. Substantial loss of myelin occurs with the disappearance of the axis cylinders. The neurolemmal sheath itself undergoes varying degrees of fibrous thickening. Hyalinization and obliteration of blood vessels causes further ischaemia of nerve fibres. The mechanism by which the damage is still not fully understood. This is, however, a rare complication, probably affecting fewer than 1% of treated clients. The most common presenting symptoms are:

- tingling and numbness of the thumb and forefinger;
- wasting and weakness of the small muscles of the hand;
- persistent pain in the shoulder region.

These symptoms appear from 6 months to over 20 years after treatment, with the most commonly reported incidence between the second and fifth year after radiotherapy. It should be emphasized that such symptoms may be caused by a variety of unrelated conditions and, if related to cancer and its treatment, are more likely to be due to recurrent cancer than RIBP.

Radiation-induced brachial plexopathy evolves: the client presents with numbness of the fingers; wasting of the small muscles of the hand will follow within months or years.

Pain will follow a variable course: characteristically it follows the distribution of nerves supplied by C5 and C6, although it may involve the whole brachial plexus. The pain varies in nature, not only in different individuals but also within the same individual at different times. Such neuropathic pain is notoriously difficult to manage.

Between one-third and two-thirds of patients with RIBP will develop progressive loss of function of the hand and arm over a period of months or years. In a minority, the condition may cease to progress without significant loss of function. In some, the severity of pain may recede as paralysis becomes complete. In others persistent pain remains.

There is a variable incidence of other associated problems including bone necrosis/fracture, lymphoedema and circulation problems. Persistent pain and increasing disability may result in clinical depression and non-specific stress-related illness.

The key to the effective management of RIBP is a collaborative multidisciplinary approach involving honest explanation and communication with both the patient and all health care professionals involved. It must be acknowledged that RIBP is essentially an incurable condition since unrealistic expectations reduce the chances of producing useful improvements in quality of life.

In the absence of definitive treatment, management should be directed towards optimizing symptom-control and function in order to maintain as good a quality of life as possible. This should be combined with careful surveillance to detect and treat recurrent cancer, particularly in the first two years after presentation.

Management involves a multidisciplinary team co-ordinated by a clinical oncologist designated in every cancer centre and cancer unit. The co-ordinating consultant oncologist is responsible for liaising with the following to make sure they are aware of protocols:

- breast-care nurse;
- physiotherapist;
- breast surgeon;
- pain clinic (anaesthetist, psychologist/psychiatrist);
- general practitioner and district nurse;
- palliative care clinic;
- occupational therapist;
- if possible, complementary therapists.

Key elements of management include:

- information and explanation to empower patients to help themselves;
- systematic management of pain;
- assistance with functions of daily living;
- psychological support including access to voluntary groups;
- regular surveillance to detect and treat cancer.

There are no hard-and-fast rules about how to help the client with RIBP as each client responds differently to treatment. The occupational therapist's input with respect to daily domestic activities can help him or her to establish a rapport with the client and this will form a basis for intervention. This input will not only cover coping with the physical disability but will also assist the client in coming to terms with disability and altered body image. The multidisciplinary team may include a specialist nurse whose role specifically includes working with altered body image, and it is important that the other health care professionals complement this work and have a similar approach. The team, therefore, needs to be co-ordinated to achieve this.

The occupational therapist may provide equipment as appropriate, for example:

- one-handed devices (for example, bread and vegetable board);
- vegetable basket for straining cooked vegetables;

- plate guard and one-handed cutlery;
- can, jar and bottle openers;
- large-handled grip on electric plug;
- suction nail brush;
- appropriate splints both for resting and dynamic use.

Spinal cord compression

Souhami and Tobias (1995) describe this syndrome as a medical emergency where treatment must begin within hours – not days – either by surgery (such as decompression laminectomy) and/or radiotherapy. The prognosis for this condition relates to the degree of neurological damage before treatment and the underlying cancer. The problem may result from the following:

- pressure on the cord, usually as a result of a tumour extending from a vertebral body and compressing the cord from the epidural space;
- direct extension from a mediastinal tumour or the cauda equina from a retroperitoneal tumour;
- a crush fracture due to weakened vertebrae;
- extradural compression developing in the absence of deposits in the spine;
- occasionally, intramedullary metastases.

It occurs most commonly in diseases with bony, particularly spinal, metastases. Cancers of the breast, prostate and lung, lymphoma and myeloma are the commonest cancers in which spinal cord compression occurs, followed by carcinomas of the thyroid, kidney, bladder, bowel and melanoma. Lymphomas may produce cord compression by extension from paraspinal lymph nodes through the intervertebral foramina.

Factors associated with spinal cord compression caused by carcinomas often include the following:

- localized back pain;
- radicular pain;
- motor deficits;
- muscle weakness;
- sensory deficits (usually seen later than motor deficits);
- parasthesias;

- decreased pain and temperature sensation;
- ataxia;
- bladder dysfunction, urinary retention, urinary dribbling;
- decreased tendon reflexes;
- paralysis – paraplegia, quadraplegia;
- loss of sphincter control.

In most cases, only one or two of these symptoms will be present and limb weakness and bladder dysfunction are late signs. Higher cord lesions will also be accompanied by symptoms and signs in the upper limbs.

When compression occurs below the lower level of the spinal cord (L1 or L2 – the cauda equina syndrome) diagnosis can be difficult as radiological investigations, including myelography, may fail to demonstrate abnormality. Compression can also occur at more than one site resulting in a mixture of upper and lower motor neurone signs.

Occupational therapy intervention requires a broad approach as cord compression will affect all aspects of the client's and carers' lives. The degree of functional impairment depends on the level of compression and success of the surgical and/or radiological treatment. The multidisciplinary team aims, therefore, for optimum functional independence but needs to be flexible in its approach. The experience of the loss of physical function also results in loss of self-esteem, a changed role within the family, and reduced economic and social status.

The early stages, resulting in localized back pain and radicular pain, may limit functional activities (putting on shoes, standing during an activity, walking). The psychological effects of pain (depression, fear of mobilizing, tension, lack of sleep, and anxiety) will increase lethargy and fatigue. Occupational therapy intervention is, therefore, required in advising and teaching alternative methods of carrying out tasks to minimize pain. Anxiety management may be appropriate to enable clients to control their feelings as well as to assist them to understand the condition and to adapt to the change in functional independence.

In order to restore the clients' confidence and self-esteem, a regular treatment programme is required. This gives structure to their day and helps the family and carers understand the aims of rehabilitation. By timetabling activities, incorporating energy conservation and avoiding situations that exacerbate the condition, clients can organize their own day to suit their needs.

Motor and sensory deficits, including anaesthesia or parasthesia of the trunk or lower limbs, present in leg weakness, loss of muscle power and atrophy, and foot-drop due to lack of dorsiflexion. Other problems include reduced balance and equilibrium reactions, ataxia, reduced co-ordination and muscle spasms. There may be potential problems of pressure areas breaking down and contractures. The resulting immobility requires the occupational therapist to fully assess and evaluate his or her role as the client responds to treatment. This depends on the individual's dysfunction. The client might initially require assistance to allow him or her to move about in bed – for example, a monkey pole, a mattress variator or a rope ladder, but continual reassessment is needed as the dysfunction changes or improves. It may be necessary for the patient to wear foot-drop splints when at rest to prevent contractures, and the physiotherapist must provide ankle/foot orthosis to aid walking. If a wheelchair is required, the arm-rests must be removable and great care should be taken when considering the means of transfer. As the client's immune system is compromised by disease and treatment, there is likely to be a very high risk of pressure areas breaking down. Even though independent transfers should be the aim, if the sacral and buttock areas are broken, hoisting must be considered.

Other transfers (including transfers in and out of bed, on and off of a commode, chair, wheelchair or WC, and in and out of a car) all need to be taught and practised daily. This will assist the carers and increase the client's self-confidence.

Self-care activities require full occupational therapy assessment in both upper and lower limb dysfunction. The individual's problems should be discussed with the client and carers in order to establish the level of outside care to be involved (for example, home care, nursing – district nursing or private). If the client and carers wish to conserve their energies for other aspects of their daily lives, their wishes must be respected. This could help prevent the social situation breaking down due to the carer being exhausted. If, however, they do not want outside intervention once the client is back at home, their wishes must also be respected.

Safety factors to be considered in activities of daily living and mobility include whether:

- the client has adequate balance to manage with a bathboard or seat;
- the steps for the accommodation are capable of being ramped safely;

- the client is safe in the kitchen, particularly when using the kettle and preparing meals and with respect to the heights of work surfaces;
- if employment is affected, the social worker should be involved regarding benefits and other appropriate intervention. If a return to work is feasible, the occupational therapist should consult with the client and employer to facilitate necessary arrangements. These may include adaptations both in terms of changes to the client's environment and in terms of workload management.
- The role of occupational therapy in leisure is particularly important. Occupational therapy in day care can be of help here (see Chapter 10).

Advice on driving may be required and this issue should be referred to the local Mobility Centre, which can provide advice on adaptations for driving. As the occupational therapist working in a general hospital is unlikely to have extensive knowledge of what is available, an information sheet can be provided by the Mobility Centre itself. Appendix 6 provides an example.

Emotional and psychological support is given as treatment progresses. This occurs over a course of time as rapport and trust is established. Counselling techniques are always employed during treatment sessions, but it is inaccurate to refer to a clinician's input as 'counselling' as this is a specific role and skill in itself. Unless the occupational therapist has trained further in the field of counselling, it is not an area in which he or she should dabble.

Dyspnoea

Difficulty in breathing is a symptom in about 30% of clients (Dunlop, 1989). It often limits exercise tolerance and levels of stamina and can be associated with increased coughing and sputum production.

Kaye (1994) describes the incidence in palliative care as

> 50% of hospice patients having dyspnoea on exertion and 75% of those with lung and pleural involvement.

However, severe dyspnoea at most occurs in only 5%. Amongst the many causes are:

- primary lung cancer;
- pulmonary metastases resulting in pleural effusion;
- radiation pneumonitis – an oedematous reaction in the tissues in response to irradiation, resulting in worsening of symptoms (for example, dyspnoea in clients with superior vena cava obstruction);

- side effects of chemotherapy;
- fluid retention (in hormone therapy for prostate cancer) causing cardiac failure.

The difficulty can be gradual in onset so the client may have become steadily debilitated. Smits (1989) observes that the client is likely to present with weight loss and sleep disturbance due to cough and so may appear more acutely ill and distressed than other groups of cancer clients. Dysfunction will present in varying degrees from minimal disability to maximum dependency. The individual needs full assessment so that areas of dysfunction can be identified. The main points for the occupational therapist to consider are:

- pressure care needs;
- placing the commode by the bed or moving the bed nearer to an accessible WC;
- help with personal care;
- correct positioning – for example, using the back rest, rope ladder and the mattress variator;
- providing equipment to enable the patient to keep exertion to a minimum, for example, a wheelchair, hydraulic bath lift, mattress variator;
- energy conservation techniques and prioritizing the daily routine;
- relaxation techniques and anxiety management.

As in all treatment programmes, the client's priorities need to be established. They should consider whether bathing or showering is an area with which they wish to continue (bathing aids are discussed in Chapter 3).

The multidisciplinary team needs to have a consistent yet flexible approach to ensure that the client maintains independence with maximum comfort and minimum anxiety. The nursing and medical teams arrange medication as well as providing psychological support together with the other team members. The physiotherapist's expertise is needed to maximize existing lung function and mobility, and the speech and language therapist is involved – particularly if there is dysphagia. If the client is cachexic, dietetic referral is very important. Dyspnoea results in decreased appetite and difficulty in finishing a full meal so nutritional advice is required.

Dyspnoea can be a frightening symptom and the occupational therapist may need to assess the home situation to advise on equipment and on the layout of strategic living areas. This can be carried out either with or without the client being present depending on whether the client is an inpatient or outpatient and on how advanced the symptoms are. It will need to be addressed as a matter of urgency.

Summary

The problem-solving approach to occupational therapy does not provide a set answer for an individual's problems. When an occupational therapist is faced with a client with spinal cord compression, for example, there is no check-list to tick off to tell him or her what to do. It may be necessary to:

- reflect on the issues discussed in Chapter 2;
- be aware of the background to the disease – not only the diagnosis but the treatment too;
- appreciate issues the client and carers are facing;
- use core psychological and physical occupational therapy skills.

When selecting the appropriate occupational therapy intervention, the therapeutic aims and benefits to the client are the main consideration.

Action points

1. For a given diagnosis, outline the symptoms and side effects you would expect the clients in an oncology and palliative care setting to experience. What role does occupational therapy have in assisting clients to cope?
2. Having identified the occupational therapy role, what would you see as your limitations? How do you refer on to other specialists and explain this to the clients?
3. Select a dysfunction or specific symptom, carry out a literature search and examine the different professionals' input into a treatment programme.

References

Black PM, Morrow GR (1991) Anticipatory nausea and emesis: behavioural interventions. In Watson M (Ed) Cancer Patient Care: Psychological Treatment Methods. Leicester: British Psychological Society.

Cassidy S (1991) Terminal care. In Watson M (Ed) Cancer Patient Care: Psychological Treatment Methods. Leicester: British Psychological Society.

Dealey C (1995) Foreword. In Waterlow J (Ed) Pressure Sore Prevention Manual. Taunton: JA Waterlow.

Dunlop GM (1989). A study of the relative frequency and importance of gastrointestinal symptoms and weakness in patients with far advanced cancer: a student paper. Palliative Medicine 4(1): 37–43.

Equipment for Disabled People (1989) Clothing and Dressing. Oxford: The Disability Information Trust.

Equipment for Disabled People (1993) Wheelchairs. Oxford: The Disability Information Trust.

Jones E (1978) Nursing patients having cancer surgery. In Borley D (Ed) Oncology for Nurses and Health Care Professionals, Volume 3. London: Harper & Row.

Kaye P (1994) A–Z of Hospice and Palliative Medicine. Northampton: EPL Publications.

Lloyd C, Coggles L (1988) Contribution of occupational therapy to pain management in cancer patients with metastatic breast disease. The American Journal of Hospice Care 5(6): 36–8.

Merton and Sutton NHS Trust Wheelchair Service (1996) Pressure Relieving Cushion Assessment. London: Merton and Sutton NHS Trust Wheelchair Service.

National Council for Hospice and Specialist Palliative Care Services (1994) Guidelines for Managing Cancer Pain in Adults. London: NCHSPCS.

Payne R (1995) Relaxation Techniques. Edinburgh: Churchill Livingstone.

Royal College of Radiologists and RAGE (1995) Guidelines on the Management of Women with Adverse Effects Following Breast Radiotherapy. London: RCR.

Smits A (1989) Nursing patients with lung cancer. In Borley D (Ed) Oncology for Nurses and Health Care Professionals, Volume 3. London: Harper & Row.

Souhami R, Tobias J (1995) Cancer and its Management. Oxford: Blackwell Scientific Publications.

Spiegel D, Bloom JR (1983) Pain in metastatic breast cancer. Cancer 52: 341–5.

Turk DC, Fernandez E (1991) Pain: a cognitive-behavioural perspective. In Watson M (Ed) Cancer Patient Care: Psychosocial Treatment Methods. Leicester: BPS.

Waterlow J (1995) Pressure Sore Prevention Manual. Taunton: JA Waterlow.

Chapter 5
Occupational Therapy in Fatigue and Energy Conservation

Jill Cooper

Fatigue involves weariness, weakness, exhaustion and lack of energy. It can be caused by exertion or stress and it results in increased discomfort and reduced efficiency, possibly affecting mental and physical activities. Dunlop (1989) lists it as the most common factor in advanced cancer, occuring in 82% of clients. Kaye (1994) advises that a careful history is needed when clients exhibit this symptom as weakness can be due to pain, lethargy or dyspnoea and must be treated appropriately.

In occupational therapy, the solution depends on a thorough history being taken in order to identify the underlying problem. For example, a referral may be received for a client who is having difficulties getting up and down the stairs. If fatigue is due to arm or leg weakness, a rail might help. If, however, it is due to dyspnoea, the rail will not provide a solution and the difficulty will be resolved by the client not attempting the stairs.

When fatigue is generalized, it is often due to spread of malignant disease. Kaye (1994) lists reversible causes of generalized weakness as:

- poor sleep;
- infection;
- anaemia;
- drugs (hypotensives, baclofen);
- hypercalcaemia;
- hypokalaemia (diuretics, steroids);
- Parkinson's disease;
- diabetes mellitus;
- hypothyroidism.

When fatigue is localized, it may be caused by:

- brain metastases;
- spinal cord compression (affecting legs);
- malignant nerve damage;
- peripheral neuropathy (foot drop, occasionally sensory loss of glove/stocking distribution);
- nerve palsy (wrist drop).

Kaye points out further areas of potential fatigue. Poor positioning can create pressure on the inside of the arm causing radial nerve palsy, or ulnar nerve palsy may occur if unpadded arm rests press on the elbow. In the case of radial nerve damage, the occupational therapist will have to provide dynamic splinting to assist the return of functioning. The occupational therapist will also have to advise on one-handed activities during the period of functional return and assess and provide equipment to assist in activities of daily living with decreased hand function.

Any assessment needs to take into consideration the stamina level of the client. A cognitive assessment such as Chessington Occupational Therapy Neurological Assessment Battery (COTNAB) might be too long and tiring to undertake in its fullest form and the occupational therapist will have to be selective in the choice of assessment, taking account of how much the client can tolerate. Advice on energy conservation is provided in Appendix 7.

Prolonged or chronic fatigue

Chronic fatigue is particularly distressing for the clients with cancer and undergoing palliative care. It is disruptive to their routine and creates physiological and psychological difficulties which, in turn, are exacerbated by external factors. Mental and physical stress experienced by carers and family causes the client to become distressed which adds to fatigue. Aistars (1987) proposed that prolonged stress results in long-standing fatigue in the client with cancer. As fatigue continues without relief, it affects functional independence and safety. General weakness is significant when it affects the client's lifestyle including his or her well-being, activities of daily living, hobbies and activities of importance to the client, and relationships and roles. Aistars (1987) lists factors contributing to chronic fatigue in cancer patients and emphasizes that the interaction of these variables ultimately determines what responses the stressors cause.

Physiological factors involve:

- cumulative effects of chemotherapy, radiotherapy or tumours;
- cumulative effects of active tumour growth, infection, fever or surgery;
- competition for nutrients between the body and the tumour;
- the cumulative effects of anorexia, nausea, vomiting, diarrhoea, constipation and bowel obstruction;
- chronic pain;
- dyspnoea;
- and anaemia.

Psychological factors may include anxiety, depression, grief, antici-patory nausea and vomiting. Other factors may involve lack of sleep, feelings of loss, immobility, relationships and the side effects of drugs. Fatigue can present with the following symptoms (Rhoten, 1982):

- *General appearance.* Pallor. Respiration is shallow. Facial muscula-ture is relaxed, and there is decreased smiling.
- *Attitude.* Flat effect, irritability, tearfulness, there is decreased moti-vation and interest.
- *Speech.* Slow monosyllabic responses or reluctant communication.
- *Activity.* Reduced performance in physical and mental activities.
- *Cognition.* Poor attention and concentration, slow and impaired perception.
- *Tiredness.* Excessive sleep or difficulty in sleeping, no energy.

The multidisciplinary team needs to plan ongoing care to support the client. An individual's needs will vary depending on his or her circumstances and support should ideally be made ready as and when required. Health care professionals should not intervene in the social situation too soon as this will take away control from the client but support should be available when needed.

It may be difficult to establish which problems result from fatigue and which arise from the disease itself. The occupational therapist is likely to have to deal with symptoms of fatigue as they arise – for example, difficulties in transfers or anxiety.

The client with advanced cancer or in palliative care is not likely to return to his or her earlier level of functioning, nor is an exercise routine likely to help build up stamina levels. Physiotherapy referral is, therefore, essential to ensure that optimum mobility is achieved and the team's approach is biased towards adaptation in the practical sense together with advice and education regarding energy conservation and stress management. Dietetic and nutritional advice is necessary to maintain energy levels, and pain control by medical and nursing staff must be established. The team needs a consistent approach to reassure the client and carers that although fatigue may be a chronic disability with which they will have to cope, there are areas of help available. This prevents them struggling to achieve a return to the previous level of function when this is not attainable.

Aistars (1987) writes that health care professionals:

- help clients recognize the condition;
- provide positive encouragement by acknowledging limitations yet offering solutions;
- provide support through active listening;
- explore emotional stressors and facilities for support;
- work with client and carers to identify their stamina levels and what level of help is most suitable for them;
- provide ongoing support;
- provide referrals for psychological support for family and carers as well as the client.

Blesch (1991) states:

> The correlation between pain and fatigue may not be independent of mood . . . there appear to be multifaceted intercorrelations between pain, mood and fatigue that may be difficult to disentangle. . . . Fatigue may be more of a problem for people who can be expected to live with their disease longer.

Social role functioning

Ricker et al. (1992) looked at perceptions of quality of life and quality of care for patients with cancer receiving chemotherapy. They confirmed previously mentioned factors which can contribute to distressing symptoms including fatigue:

- tension/anxiety, depression/dejection, anger/hostility, vigour/activity, fatigue/inertia, confusion/bewilderment;
- mood, level of anxiety;
- well-being, pain, nausea and appetite;
- level of physical activity, ability to perform job-related duties or housework and social activities;

- the impact of cancer on the quality of the client's relationship with his or her spouse;
- change in level of satisfaction.

They found that: 'Social role functioning was linked positively to perceived quality of life.' Some patients reported strain on relationships adding to the stress and hence fatigue, whilst others reported that the disease stengthened their bond. Significant factors that were of great comfort to the clients and carers were adequate symptom control, communication with the multidisciplinary team, and adequate information about how care was proceeding. Pickard-Holley (1991) described a study examining relationships between fatigue and various physical and psychological factors in women undergoing chemotherapy for ovarian cancer:

> In the person with cancer . . . fatigue is a concern at many points during the disease process and treatment, and the problem is not easily resolved by a brief rest period or a good night's sleep. Persons with cancer describe a variety of problems, e.g. tiredness, lack of energy, generalized lassitude, inability to sustain exertion, loss of motor power, impaired mobility, sleepiness, drowsiness, confusion, apathy, poor concentration, helplessness, a sense of inadequacy and an inability to mobilize energy to carry on.

Fatigue has adverse effects on well-being, daily living, valued relationships and compliance with treatment. It is, therefore, important to incorporate advice on living with fatigue into occupational therapy programmes.

Cancer clients experience a significant increase in fatigue over a 5- or 6-week course of radiotherapy and 14 days after treatment with chemotherapy. Fatigue gradually diminishes but does remain 3 months after treatment has finished in a small percentage of clients. Fatigue following radiotherapy may also be related to weight loss, negative mood and pain. This may further affect functional independence and relationships, such stresses adding to fatigue (Irvine *et al.*, 1994).

Clients need to look at how their daily routine is spread out by:

- having a weekly diary or timetable;
- making priorities and choices;
- shedding those activities with which they cannot/do not wish to continue;
- organizing tasks, visitors, etc. to suit their own stamina level;

- ensuring that if they are tired after 20 minutes, they just work for 15 minutes and rest. This is to avoid fatigue.

Clients may find visitors very tiring and feel guilty if someone has gone to the trouble of visiting them. However, it is important that friends and family understand how exhausted the client becomes and time limits should be put on their stay.

Physiological influences

In helping the client adjust to fatigue, the occupational therapist needs to be aware of how the disease and treatment create this distressing symptom.

Regnard and Mannix (1992) state that:

> The words drowsiness, tiredness, lethargy, fatigue and weakness have different meanings to different patients. Drowsiness usually means an impairment of cognition such as the reduced alertness caused by sedative drugs.

Kaye (1994) lists reversible causes of fatigue, including drugs. When drugs cause fatigue, the solution is to reduce or change the dose or the drug. Anaemia contributes to tiredness and fatigue, particularly if the haemoglobin is below 9 g/dl. Motor weakness affecting skeletal muscle is usually localized in a muscle or in groups of muscles. If spinal cord compression occurs, surgical decompression and/or radiotherapy is required and occupational therapy intervention is covered in Chapter 4.

Regnard and Mannix (1992) observe that enabling clients to take frequent rest periods will help them to conserve energy. By careful planning, frustration will be avoided and positive benefits of these rest periods will be reinforced. Again, appropriate mobility training, nutritional advice and spiritual and psychological care is needed for clients to achieve global well-being.

St Pierre et al. (1992) state that 'the specific mechanisms underlying cancer fatigue are unclear.' Dysfunction relating to the skeletal muscle is suggested as clients:

- often develop skeletal muscle wasting as part of cancer cachexia accompanied by fatigue;
- cytokines such as tumour necrosis factor (TNF) that are used to treat cancers are known to be associated with fatigue, leading to metabolic changes in skeletal muscle;

- exercise used in cancer rehabilitation can induce fatigue by altering concentration of skeletal muscle metabolites.

Any exercise in individuals with advanced cancer must be moderate and must have clear treatment aims and objectives – such as enabling the client to continue to manage stairs. As energy stores are depleted and the body has no opportunity to restore this energy, the client has to cope with this stress on a continual basis, resulting in fatigue (Blesch *et al.*, 1991). Bruera and MacDonald (1988) suggest:

> a primary mechanism of fatigue may be structural or functional abnormalities in muscle tissue, possibly brought about by a substance(s) produced by the tumour.

Research has suggested that malnutrition, cachexia and infection in people with cancer may be part of such mechanisms.

Haylock and Hart (1979) listed complications accompanying 'localized radiation' as: 'weakness, extreme tiredness, headache, nausea and vomiting, diarrhoea, rectal irritation, anorexia, dry mouth, skin irritation and/or breakdown.' Fatigue among clients receiving radiotherapy may be due to the body's inability to maintain an equilibrium when stressors place demands on homeostatic mechanisms. They quote Cannon's (1932) theory, which suggests that the body is reserving energy to repair itself after therapy, and another unproven theory that fatigue is caused by the accumulation of end products of destroyed cells and toxicities inhibiting normal cell function. Clinicians have noted that the absence of exposure to radiotherapy over weekends is consistently followed by reduced fatigue levels. The occupational therapist can therefore help the client capitalize on times when they are feeling least tired by timetabling routines and including regular rests and breaks.

Sexuality

Fatigue is likely to be a major factor in difficulties with sexuality. Whether the underlying problems relating to dysfunction are physical or psychological, the client needs to be able to discuss these. Unless a health care professional has a close rapport and has time to give to the individual, it is unlikely that the client will raise the subject. The occupational therapist may be able to discuss the client's worries and, if further advice is needed, refer the matter to the appropriate specialist.

Physical problems may be due to pain following surgery, or to side effects of treatment such as chemotherapy or endocrine therapy. Such side effects may include vaginal dryness. Once the physical discomfort has become a problem, this in turn creates anxiety and the client begins to dread intercourse. Advice needs to be sought on changing the medication or overcoming the side effects.

The underlying problem might be altered body image. This can be worked through by discussing fears or referring on to a specialist. All these factors can combine to cause clients to worry about their sexuality and this may exacerbate the fatigue.

The occupational therapist can look at the structure of the day and establish whether it is possible for clients to take a rest in order to be able to carry on with their sexual relationships. Many clients find they experience fatigue for up to two years after radiotherapy and if the partner finds it difficult to understand why the fatigue is continuing, they may need to discuss what each wants out of the relationship. Communicating these worries and fears may avoid misunderstanding and the breakdown of relationships. Advice on sexual functioning may be needed from a specialist if problems relate to specific gynaecological cancers, and referral to a counsellor may be necessary if relationships are severely affected.

Case study

Name: Mrs A

Age: 47

Diagnosis: Widespread metastatic carcinoma of right breast, originally diagnosed four years earlier. Metastases affecting lungs, left eye and liver.

Past medical history: Four years ago seen in clinic with ulcerated right breast. Reported she had been aware of changes to breast for four years and complained of visual blurring.

Four years ago metastatic area of left eye treated with radiotherapy.

Seen six-monthly by breast unit.

Treatment: palliative radiotherapy.

Social history: Retired schoolteacher for people with learning difficulties. Lives alone, separated from husband with whom she has no contact. Two grown children (son and daughter) and grandchildren, live locally, very supportive.

Social support: Two very good neighbours, sees district nurse twice a week to dress ulcerated breast.

Presenting problems/symptoms:

- exhaustion upon exertion;
- extreme shortness of breath;
- requires assistance from one person to mobilize;
- inability to complete personal care independently;
- inability to carry out domestic activities independently.

Aims of occupational therapy intervention:

- To enable Mrs A to structure and pace tasks allowing for fluctuating energy and breathing levels and likelihood of reduced stamina.
- To facilitate Mrs A's independence in transfers.
- To enable Mrs A to achieve a level of mobility that gives her independence over short distances.
- To enable Mrs A to meet personal care needs.
- To ensure Mrs A has her domestic needs met.
- To enable Mrs A opportunities to discuss any concerns she is experiencing.

Objectives of occupational therapy intervention:

- Mrs A will establish an ability to break down tasks into components to reserve energy and minimize shortness of breath.
- The occupational therapist will identify optimum furniture heights to facilitate Mrs A's independence.
- Mrs A will establish own level of walking ability and tolerance.
- The occupational therapist and Mrs A will identify precise problem areas of personal activities of daily living. With Mrs A's permission, the level and type of assistance will be noted and appropriate community services requested to help.
- Mrs A and the occupational therapist will identify realistic needs for domestic input following daily living and mobility assessments.
- The occupational therapist and Mrs A will build a rapport so that she will feel able to express any feeling and thoughts of anxiety and concerns.

Occupational therapy intervention

Whilst an inpatient, Mrs A was assessed in personal activities of daily living. Daily practice established areas in which she felt she could manage and areas in which she felt she would benefit from assistance. By building up rapport and trust, Mrs A realized that she could allow others to help her, she acknowledged her own limitations and she gave herself permission to ask for input from health care professionals.

During treatment sessions, Mrs A was able to look objectively at her daily routine and plan her time to avoid becoming overtired.

Assessment and treatment with physiotherapist enabled Mrs A to walk, making the most efficient use of her energy levels, and to control breathing. She was encouraged to take regular rests.

Home assessment was carried out without Mrs A, prior to her discharge from hospital, to take measurements of furniture heights, and to arrange for provision of furniture raisers to enable safe transfers and conserve energy.

Because of her complex needs, Mrs A was able to meet with the multidisciplinary team members individually and as a group in a case conference. She was not intimidated by this because she knew everyone and was pleased to talk to them. Thus a co-ordinated discharge package was planned with her agreement and her contributions as well as those of the team. This gave her back an element of control over the situation despite her failing health and reassured her that she could contact any member of the team if any further concerns were raised. After alleviating the physical obstacles as far as possible, and reducing her concerns regarding coping, her fatigue was observed to be less severe.

Summary

Clients are likely to experience spells of fatigue in the acute as well as the advanced stages of disease. It is extremely frustrating for them to lose control over their life and not be able to function at the premorbid level. Many clients express guilt at not being able to manage the same workload, whether it is domestic or paid work. The occupational therapist can provide advice on energy conservation, practical tips, and permission to slow down and adjust their standards to what is realistic. The client may need to negotiate the workload with the employer if he or she cannot achieve the same output. Similarly, there may be a need for negotiation with the family concerning what is expected in the home.

By deciding which activities are important to the client, perhaps grading them from 1 to 5, the client and the occupational therapist can work together to make a list of those with which the client wants to continue and those which can be given up.

Fatigue is a challenging symptom for the occupational therapist. In order to be realistic, the approach needs to be flexible so that the client can cope with whatever demands are being made. The client's level of motivation needs to be assessed as this will influence his or her functional performance, and the occupational therapist needs to be aware of other factors causing weariness and lethargy.

References

Aistars J (1987) Fatigue in the cancer patient: a conceptual approach to a clinical problem. Oncology Nursing Forum 14(6): 25–30.

Blesch K, Paice JA, Wickham R, Harte N, Schnoor DK, Purl S, Rehwalt M, Lam Kopp P, Manson S, Coveny SB, McHale M, Cahill M (1991) Correlates of fatigue in people with breast or lung cancer. Oncology Nursing Forum 14(6): 17–23.

Bruera E, MacDonald RN (1988) Asthenia in patients with advanced cancer. Journal of Pain Symptom Management 3(1): 9–14.

Dunlop GM (1989) A study of the relative frequency and importance of gastrointestinal symptoms and weakness in patients with far advanced cancer: a student paper. Palliative Medicine 4: 37–43.

Haylock PJ, Hart LK (1979) Fatigue in patients receiving localized radiation. Cancer Nursing 2: 461–7.

Irvine DM, Vincent L, Graydon J, Bubela N, Thompson L (1991) A critical approach to the research literature investigating fatigue in the individual with cancer. Cancer Nursing 14(1): 188–99.

Kaye P (1994) A–Z of Hospice and Palliative Medicine. Northampton: EPL Publications.

McCorkle R, Young K (1978) Development of a symptom distress scale. Cancer Nursing 1: 373–8.

Pickard-Holley S (1991) Fatigue in cancer patients. A descriptive study. Cancer Nursing 14(1): 13–19.

Piper BF, Lindsey AM, Dodd MJ (1987) Fatigue mechanisms in cancer patients: developing nursing theory. Oncology Nursing Forum 14(6): 17–23.

Regnard C, Mannix K (1992) Weakness and fatigue in advanced cancer – a flow diagram. Palliative Medicine 6: 253–6.

Rhoten D (1982) Fatigue and the postsurgical patient. In Norris CM (Ed) Concept Clarification in Nursing. Rockville, MD: Aspen Publishers Inc. pp. 277–300.

Rieker PP, Clark EJ, Fogelberg PR (1992) Perceptions of quality of life and quality of care for patients with cancer receiving biological therapy. Oncology Nursing Forum 19(3): 433–40.

St Pierre BA, Kasper CE, Lindsey AM (1992) Fatigue mechanisms in patients with cancer: effects of tumour necrosis factor and exercise on skeletal muscle. Oncology Nursing Forum 19(3): 419–25.

Chapter 6
Occupational Therapy in Stress and Anxiety Management

Gillian McVey

It can be stressful to experience the physical and psychological changes associated with cancer and its treatment. Significant anxiety or depression is found in 25% of clients with advanced cancer (Kaye, 1994). To deal with such a diagnosis, clients have to learn to live as productively as possible.

Stress management offers one way in which occupational therapists can address the physical and psychological needs of those with cancer, at any stage of the disease process. This chapter discusses the reasons for stress and anxiety in those with cancer together with the theory of stress management and its application in oncology.

Stress and cancer

A cancer diagnosis will start a rapid process of adjustment which will involve alterations in lifestyle and extensive role changes. Mehls (1983) stated that 'the patient with cancer is often overwhelmed by the global effects of the disease on himself and his family.' These relentless feelings of losing control may be experienced at any stage of the disease process. The following factors may cause stress for the individual diagnosed with cancer:

* the serious and potentially life-threatening nature of this illness;
* possible uncertainty regarding the cause of cancer, its diagnosis, prognosis, the length and nature of treatment and its side effects;
* fear of pain;
* fear of helplessness and increasing physical and psychological dependence on others;

- adapting to changes in body image such as mastectomy, hair loss, weight loss, lymphoedema and skin changes due to radiation;
- confronting issues of death and dying.

All these issues can lead to feelings of stress. Lazarus (1971) defined stress as:

> a broad class of problems differentiated from other problem areas, because it deals with any demands which tax the system . . . physiological . . . social . . . psychological systems and the response of that system.

The stress response depends on the unconscious or conscious appraisal of a 'harmful, threatening or challenging event'. The level of stress experienced depends on the level of emotional support available, personality factors, how the diagnosis is perceived by clients, their previous experiences and perceptions of cancer, and cultural factors. Informal carers may also experience a degree of stress and lifestyle change, so they may not be able to provide emotional support consistently.

The psychological problems experienced by the individual with cancer can be varied. They may depend on the level of disruption to the roles and expectations the individual holds. Disruption, leading to symptoms of stress, may be more apparent when the disease appears to be progressing, at the onset of side effects of treatment, and if clients are experiencing discordant attitudes from others towards the cancer and its treatment. Throughout the course of the disease, there will be increasing role changes for the client and the carers. These may be of a physical, social or financial nature.

Stress is a common experience and often occurs whether one has a cancer diagnosis or not. For some, stress provides new challenges and can be a positive experience resulting in change; for others it can produce negative physical and psychological results.

Anxiety

Anxiety is a normal biological defence mechanism that warns the body of potential danger and allows it to react quickly in times of stress. A degree of anxiety with resulting muscular tension is normal; it serves to motivate and stimulate individuals to act or respond to daily situations. Feelings of stress may occur when there has been a threat to one's identity as discussed previously – for example, a change in status with a resulting change in role, commonly seen in the individual with cancer. The stress may occur before the individual is able to adapt to the new situation, either behaviourally or psychologically. The individual is not in control and this increasing lack of control can lead to anxiety. The ability to cope will be decreased if no apparent changes in behaviour can alleviate the anxiety and if the stress is excessive in duration and intensity. Such stress can result in reduced energy, initiative and motivation over a prolonged period and possibly other physical complaints.

The anxiety response

The human body has evolved over millions of years yet it still retains basic responses that were more useful to the ancestors of mankind. One such response is the 'fight-or-flight' response: the desire to attack or run away when faced with a threatening stimulus.

The 'fight-or-flight' response involves the hormone adrenaline being released into the bloodstream to increase the heart rate and improve blood flow, and increased respiration to allow more oxygen to reach the circulatory system. This improves the blood supply to the voluntary muscles, which become tensed for action.

All the above reactions can result in:

- increased activity;
- production of heat and water;
- increased flushing and sweating;
- improved blood supply to voluntary muscles;
- a sinking, nauseous feeling in the stomach
- evacuation of bowel and bladder to reduce body weight.

If an individual meets a challenging or potentially dangerous or stressful situation, the 'fight-or-flight' response will prove useful as it can improve performance. The response can, however, also occur in a safe situation which should offer security and hope – for example, when attending hospital for chemotherapy. Although the fear is understandable to a certain degree, it can become irrational and out of control. If this happens several times, unproductive lasting muscle activity may be triggered and can result in increased stress.

Suppose, for example, Ms W has recently been diagnosed with breast cancer and has to attend the outpatient clinic at her local hospital for a course of chemotherapy. Following her first chemotherapy session, she experiences a degree of nausea and vomiting – common side effects of her particular regime. As her second appointment approaches, she begins to feel nauseous even before she leaves her home; her anxiety increases and so, in turn, does the nausea. She begins to lose confidence regarding her ability to cope with six more sessions of chemotherapy and when she reaches the hospital she is extremely anxious and begins to wonder whether she can face going for this chemotherapy session. This in turn can lead to a sense of failure and increasing anxiety-related symptoms. It then starts to become difficult for her to distinguish between anxiety symptoms and side effects of chemotherapy. If she is unable to modify the above reaction, it is likely to continue and worsen. On subsequent visits to the hospital her reaction may become an anxiety spiral.

The anxiety spiral

Awareness of how physical symptoms can occur in an anxiety-provoking situation can often bring about those symptoms in that situation. This may be anticipatory or evoked by the memory of a past experience. Often there is a feeling that there is something

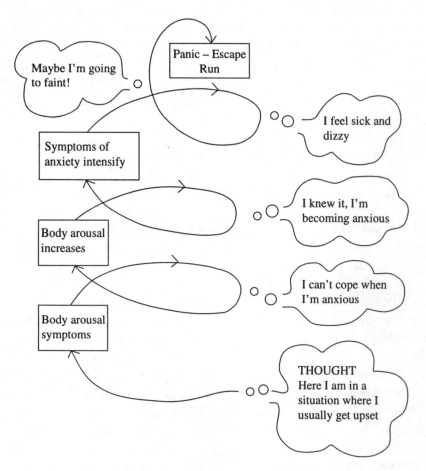

Figure 6.1: The anxiety spiral

wrong with bodily functions and this increases the tension and exacerbates the symptoms. The result is the 'anxiety spiral' which can culminate in panic and the desire to run away. The situation that evoked the feelings remains and needs to be addressed.

By using cognitive behavioural techniques, such as relaxation or positive thinking, one may cut through the anxiety spiral and stop its cumulative effects. The benefits of feeling at ease may be noticed and the anxiety will hopefully subside, allowing the situation to be addressed more effectively.

Anxiety symptoms

A variety of physical and psychological symptoms can result from anxiety and stress. Each individual will react to anxiety-provoking situations in his or her own way and is unlikely to experience all the symptoms listed. The reasons for these bodily changes will be discussed in greater depth later. The symptoms might include the following:

Physical symptoms

- tense muscles;
- excessive fatigue;
- tension headaches;
- palpitations;
- dizziness;
- blackouts;
- stomach churning;
- tightness in throat and chest;
- restlessness;
- excessive sweating;
- shaking;
- stammering.

Psychological symptoms

- apprehension;
- insomnia;
- loss of confidence;
- depression;
- short temper;
- irritability;
- self-consciousness;

- sexual difficulties;
- fears;
- phobias;
- difficulty in personal relationships;
- difficulty in formulating thoughts.

Trigger points for muscular tension

When faced with a stressful situation, some areas of the body may become more tense than others. These are *trigger points*. Common areas include:

- forehead – excessive frowning;
- shoulders – hunched up and forward;
- hands clenching – wringing, clasping;
- lower back – pain and discomfort;
- neck – pain;
- legs – cramps, muscular pain;
- chest – pain.

If individuals can be taught to recognize their own trigger points for muscular tension, steps can be taken to concentrate on relaxing it as soon as the area is triggered by the anxiety. This may stop anxiety levels rising, allow the whole body to become relaxed, and cause the situation to be defused. If muscle groups are continually triggered by anxiety, the results can be unproductive fixed activity and a change in posture.

Stress management

Clients should be made aware of the need to take personal responsibility for managing their own stress outside occupational therapy sessions. The effectiveness of stress management will largely depend on their willingness to change, their level of insight into maladaptive responses and their motivation to develop adaptive coping strategies. Depending on the resources available in the occupational therapy department and the numbers and diagnoses of those referred for stress management, the therapist needs to decide whether to offer individual and/or open or closed group sessions. The therapist also needs to decide the format of a programme. It should aim to assist clients with cancer to gain a greater understanding of their stress response in terms of its origin, course and nature. It should aim to offer a practical way to change maladaptive responses in order to restore control over the environment. This intervention consists of two main components:

- cognitive, and
- physiological.

Cognitive component of stress management

The cognitive element is based on the theory that maladaptive responses arise from a distortion of thoughts. Negative emotions can arise from the interpretation of events the individual actually experiences or expects to experience. The danger of situations is often irrationally overestimated. Beck (1989) discussed how anxiety and the resulting stress arise from a repeated distortion of danger or a tendency to view performance in a negative manner. This has four main dimensions:

- Overestimating the chances of a feared event occurring.
- Overestimating the severity of that event.
- Underestimating the ability to cope with such an event.
- Underestimating the potential of external assistance for the above.

Once these thought processes start:

- The individual becomes stressed.
- He or she expects failure or disaster.
- He or she begins to look out for other sources of stress.
- The individual finds that he or she is unable to function due to the anxiety attack.

This is demonstrated in the anxiety spiral. Beck (1989) states that the longer this dysfunctional behaviour continues, the greater is the likelihood that the individual will develop errors in cognition processes such as:

- Anticipating danger and predicting the outcome in negative terms.
- Exaggerating minor mistakes as total failure.
- Overgeneralizing by concentrating on negative experiences as the basis for existence and being.
- Ignoring his or her positive qualities by rejecting strengths, gains and personal resources to cope with stress.

As part of a stress-management programme, the techniques listed below can be utilized to modify dysfunctional behaviour and cognitive processes:

- Identifying negative thoughts.
- Understanding the meaning of negative thoughts in relation to situations.
- Challenging and modifying thoughts.
- Restructuring thoughts by the substitution of alternative interpretations and functional or positive thought patterns.
- The use of behavioural experiments such as role play and imagery.

Practice is essential for the above skills to be acquired. Gradual exposure to situations should be enforced and reviewed. The occupational therapist should enable the individual to set realistic goals in order to apply and test skills between sessions. This may also involve the application of other techniques, such as assertiveness training, time management and goal setting, in order to realistically achieve adaptive responses to stress.

Physiological component of stress management

The physiological element is based on the premise that physical, hormonal and endocrine reactions occur inappropriately as responses to threatening events. This is discussed by Powell and Enright (1991) and Madders (1988). As the individual recognizes or anticipates a feared event, the body undergoes a series of hormonal and endocrine reactions, initiated by the hypothalamus in the brain. The sympathetic nervous system prepares the body for the possibility of vigorous physical activity. This involves:

- Release of glucose from the liver.
- Increased need for oxygen as glucose is transported in the blood and transformed to energy.
- A resulting increase in heart rate and blood pressure.
- The increased demand for oxygen leads to increased respiration.
- Increased muscular tension.
- Release of adrenaline.
- Other bodily changes, such as sweating, dilated pupils and increased need to pass urine or defecate.

The above bodily changes occur rapidly and unconsciously in response to situations seen as threatening or dangerous. The methods listed below should be included as part of a stress-management programme to help modify inappropriate responses and cope with the physiological element of stress.

- Increasing awareness about physical stress responses, bodily changes and the level of arousal that can be tolerated.
- Teaching self-help methods such as breathing control and relaxation to induce physiological effects that counteract those of the stress response, and distraction to focus attention away from bodily changes.
- Facilitating lifestyle changes – for example, in nutrition, exercise, recreation and social support networks.

Application of stress management in oncology

Stress management can be beneficial in assisting the individual with cancer to achieve control over anxiety and improve his or her quality of life. Bridge *et al.* (1988) found that, by using relaxation and imagery in the treatment of breast cancer, mood improved significantly compared to those patients receiving just relaxation or no interventions. In this study, the individuals who benefited most were receiving radiotherapy for breast cancer and were aged over 55 years.

Oldham (1989) discussed the use of stress management and, in particular, the use of relaxation and guided imagery to meet the psychological needs of cancer patients. This work was considered to be most cost-effective when practised in group sessions. This was also reported by Grassman (1993), who used stress management as part of educational and support programmes for cancer patients. Unfortunately these studies did not employ experimental evaluation techniques.

Nausea and vomiting are common side effects of chemotherapy. Morrow and Hickok (1993) reported that:

> a substantial proportion of patients . . . develop these symptoms in anticipation of treatment after one or more courses of chemotherapy have been given.

For chemotherapy-related nausea and vomiting, behavioural techniques, including the use of progressive muscular relaxation, were found to be 'effective in preventing as well as decreasing these symptoms'.

Troesch *et al.* (1993) reported that guided imagery was also beneficial in assisting with the above symptoms and increasing clients' coping skills. Those who received this intervention were able to view chemotherapy as a 'significantly more positive experience'.

The value of stress management interventions in oncology settings may be dependent on diagnoses and personality factors. Edgar *et al.* (1992) used cognitive techniques and relaxation training with individuals with cancer during the first year after diagnosis. They concluded that:

> patients with low ego strength and . . . [cancer] . . . diagnoses other than breast cancer might be at higher risk for psychosocial complications and could benefit from interventions.

This highlights a need for more quantitative and qualitative research across all cancer diagnoses.

Finally, Maguire *et al.* (1993) presented a model for the practical application of cognitive and behavioural techniques in conjunction with medication to deal with anxiety in the later stages of cancer. It was emphasized that early intervention is necessary to prevent the disabling effects of a clinical anxiety state which may hinder symptom control in advanced disease.

It can be seen that several health care professionals have studied the effects of stress in cancer and the application of stress management in this clinical specialty. However, it is clear that further work on its effectiveness and practical application is required, particularly with regard to the role of the occupational therapist.

Use of relaxation

Relaxation can be used by virtually anyone, although cognitive skills should be relatively intact. It may assist in coping with feelings of anxiety and can become part of a daily routine. There are several relaxation techniques suitable for use in oncology, including progressive muscular relaxation, guided imagery and autosuggestion (Payne, 1995). It is advisable to include a variety of relaxation techniques in any programme. Clients can then select and learn the most appropriate and effective ones for their needs. Relaxation techniques should be selected on an individual basis, depending on symptoms and preferences. Those techniques that are physically based, such as progressive muscular relaxation, might not be appropriate for clients experiencing considerable bone or muscular pain. The format of tensing and relaxing muscle groups could heighten symptoms or be too difficult. Likewise, those with limited concentration or extreme fatigue may need to utilize techniques that are short in duration, but still as effective in reducing anxiety symptoms. Techniques to aid relaxation are not to be used when driving!

The occupational therapist should teach clients how to prepare for relaxation techniques:

- First, they should tell the people with whom they share their home that they will need at least 20 minutes every day to practise relaxation undisturbed. It is important to allow plenty of time for relaxation so that the session is finished slowly and gently.
- They should try to ensure there will be no distractions – for example, by animals or telephones.
- They should be comfortable and the room should be warm.
- If they choose to lie down, they should use something which is firm rather than the bed or sofa.
- Ensure that they practise as often as possible in pleasant surroundings.
- A personal stereo cassette player may be useful in reducing background distractions.

After a relaxation session:

- They should leave the imagined surroundings slowly by becoming aware of the sounds in the external environment.
- They should be aware of how relaxed they feel.
- Movement should be slow and gentle, stretching all limbs.
- They should be aware of the physical and psychological feeling of a relaxed state.

Clients with cancer should be reminded that learning relaxation techniques involves no drugs, no unpleasant side effects, no difficult postures or strenuous exercise and no 'brainwashing' or hypnosis. Clients should have an understanding of basic principles, be aware of the need to practise techniques and should try to increase their confidence in their body to adjust to stress. Understanding how relaxation can help manage anxiety may increase motivation and willingness to practise regularly. It is also important for the occupational therapist to make it clear to the client that relaxation is a skill that has to be learned and that, without regular practice, it may be difficult for some individuals to experience the results they want.

After teaching clients a relaxation technique, it may be useful to have a prerecorded tape available so they can practise at home and use the new coping skill between therapy sessions. Relaxation tapes are available commercially but those with the therapist's voice recorded on them may improve compliance as the individual will be able to identify and recall the desired response more readily. Tapes should be seen as a small part of an overall stress-management programme; they should complement therapy sessions, not replace them.

In order to assist compliance and increase motivation it may be helpful to explain the reasons for learning and using relaxation to the client. For those with cancer, the reasons may be to:

- improve quality of sleep;
- lessen pain caused by inappropriate muscle tension;
- encourage peace of mind;
- improve physical skills;
- increase self-esteem and confidence;
- ease relationships with others;
- learn a coping strategy for feelings of anxiety;
- channel and control effects of anxiety;
- avoid unnecessary fatigue;
- improve quality of life.

Relaxation can be helpful in alleviating symptoms of anxiety but needs to be incorporated with other cognitive and behavioural strategies in addressing the stress experienced by those with cancer.

Conducting stress and anxiety management

Stress management can take place on an individual or group basis, on a ward, in a client's home or in an occupational therapy department. Whatever, the location, it should be free from as much external interference as possible – it should take place in quiet surroundings with no telephones, animals or bleeps, and the room should have curtains or blinds. It is advisable to put a notice on the door to indicate that a session is taking place to avoid interruptions. Whether stress management is to take place on an individual or group basis, it is advisable to have a programme planned before sessions commence and to agree a contract block of sessions with the client. This will provide a means of reviewing the effectiveness of sessions with individuals who have been referred and enable the occupational therapist to discharge the client. There should be a clearly defined number of sessions. It should always be remembered that referral to another member of the multidisciplinary team may be appropriate in addressing the client's psychological needs.

A stress-management programme run as a closed group for women with breast cancer is discussed and evaluated by Watson *et al.* (1996). The group sessions outlined were organized and facilitated by an occupational therapist, a clinical psychologist and a clinical nurse specialist in breast cancer at an oncology centre. The six closed-group sessions took place weekly for two hours and involved 10 to 12 group members, all newly diagnosed breast cancer clients with no clinical evidence of metastatic spread. Posters around the hospital promoted the availability of these groups and referrals were taken from other professionals and the clients themselves. Those interested were individually assessed for suitability using structured interviews. Information was provided on group format and emphasis placed on members being active learners and assuming responsibility for creating change to maladaptive responses to stress. The group sessions encompassed the cognitive and physiological elements of stress and its management. There was opportunity for learning practical coping strategies, such as time management and relaxation, and rehearsal and evaluation of skills. The additional opportunity to meet with other women with breast cancer was reassuring and created a potential social support system. Other health care professionals attended a session – for example, the dietitian attended one to promote discussion on making lifestyle changes to deal with the stresses of living with breast cancer.

Another relaxation-training programme was run by the occupational therapist at the same oncology centre for those suffering from cancer who, it was felt, would benefit from it and who were willing to learn and use relaxation techniques to assist in controlling feelings of anxiety. A poster offering the service was sited throughout patient areas of the hospital. Referrals for relaxation training were accepted from all members of the multidisciplinary team, verbally or written. The referring member provided details of the client's medical condition and level of anxiety and the client was told that he or she was being referred to ensure that they were willing to participate. Self-referrals were also encouraged as this demonstrated a higher level of motivation to participate. Inpatients who were referred were usually initially seen on the ward, but training continued on an outpatient basis if this was appropriate and feasible.

Initial interview

The purpose of the initial interview was to ascertain by questioning and/or observation:

- the present level of anxiety experienced;
- its effect on daily routine;
- current treatment regimes and any side effects;
- past medical history and medication taken, and
- previous use of relaxation.

This initial assessment formed the baseline for further appropriate intervention either on an individual or group basis (see Appendix 9). The format of sessions depended on individual needs but aimed to demonstrate the use of relaxation as a means of reducing anxiety symptoms. An example of a format, for four sessions, is shown in Appendix 10.

The purpose and format of relaxation training were explained verbally to the client. A form with the aims of relaxation training was given to the client for further information with dates of individual or group sessions. The contact name and telephone number of the occupational therapist responsible for training was also given and the client was encouraged to make enquiries should problems regarding the use of relaxation be encountered. At the final session an evaluation form was issued for the individual to return anonymously to the department in a prepaid envelope, as seen in Appendix 11. Evaluation and audit of services is vital in implementing changes and planning resources.

Examples of relaxation scripts are given in Appendix 12.

Summary

From the moment of diagnosis and throughout the survival period, the individual with cancer faces many potential stressors. Recognizing these stressors and learning to deal with their effects on lifestyle and daily living may improve quality of life and the range of coping mechanisms. For occupational therapists working in oncology, stress and anxiety management and relaxation offer an invaluable and holistic intervention.

References

Beck AT (1989) Cognitive Therapy and the Emotional Disorders. Harmondsworth: Penguin.

Bridge LR, Benson P, Pietroni PC, Priest, RG (1988) Relaxation and imagery in the treatment of breast cancer. British Medical Journal 297: 1169–72.

Cox C (1988) Practical aspects of stress management. British Journal of Occupational Therapy 51(2): 44–7.

Edgar L, Rosberger Z, Nowlis D (1992) Coping with cancer during the first year after diagnosis. Assessment and intervention. Cancer 69: 817–28.

Grassman D (1993) Development of inpatient oncology educational and support programs. Oncology Nursing Forum 20(4), 669–76.

Kaye P (1994) A–Z of Hospice and Palliative Medicine. Northampton: EPL Publications.

Lazarus RS (1971) The concept of stress and disease. In Levi L (Ed) Society, Stress and Disease, Volume 1. London: Oxford University Press.

Madders J (1988) Stress and Relaxation. London: Macdonald Optima.

Maguire P, Faulkner A, Regnard C (1993) Managing the anxious patient with advancing disease – a flow diagram. Palliative Medicine 7: 239–44.

Mehls JD (1983) Occupational therapy as a component of cancer rehabilitation. In Progress of Cancer Control III: A Regional Approach. New York: Alan Liss Inc., pp. 231–40.

Morrow GR, Hickok JT (1993) Behavioural treatment of chemotherapy-induced nausea and vomiting. Oncology 7(12): 83–9.

Oldham J (1989) Psychological support for cancer patients. British Journal of Occupational Therapy 52(12): 463–5.

Payne R (1995) Relaxation Techniques. Edinburgh: Churchill Livingstone.

Powell TJ, Enright SJ (1991) Anxiety and Stress Management. London: Routledge.

Troesch, LM, Blust Rodehaver C, Delaney EA, Yanes B (1993) The influence of guided imagery on chemotherapy-related nausea and vomiting. Oncology Nursing Forum 20(8): 1179–85.

Watson M, Fenlon D, McVey G, Fernandez-Marcos M (1996) A support group for breast cancer patients: development of a cognitive-behavioural approach. Behavioural and Cognitive Psychotherapy 24: 73–81.

Further reading

Craik C (1988) Stress in occupational therapy: how to cope. British Journal of Occupational Therapy 51(2): 40–3.

Keable D (1985) Relaxation training techniques – a review. Part one: what is relaxation? British Journal of Occupational Therapy: 99–102.

Keable D (1985) Relaxation training techniques – a review. Part two: how effective is relaxation training? British Journal of Occupational Therapy: 201–4.

Lerman C, Rimer B, Blumberg B, Cristinzio S, Engstrom PF, MacElwee N, O'Connor K, Seay J (1990) Effects of coping style and relaxation on cancer chemotherapy side effects and emotional responses. Oncology Nursing Forum 13(5): 308–15.

Mastenbroek I, McGovern L (1991) The effectiveness of relaxation techniques in controlling chemotherapy induced nausea: a literature review. The Australian Occupational Therapy Journal 38(3): 137–42.

Oberst MT, Hughes SH, McCubbin MA (1991) Self care burden, stress appraisal and mood among persons receiving radiotherapy. Cancer Nursing 14(2): 71–8.

Payne R (1995) Relaxation Techniques. Edinburgh: Churchill Livingstone.

Strong J (1991) Relaxation training and chronic pain. British Journal of Occupational Therapy 54(6): 216–18.

Westland G (1988) Relaxing in primary health care. British Journal of Occupational Therapy 51(3): 84–8.

Chapter 7
Occupational Therapy in Paediatric Oncology

Shona Bruce Crosthwaite

Very little has been published on the role of the occupational therapist in the care of patients with cancer (Picard and Magno, 1982;
Whitley, Branscomb and Moreno, 1979; Dudgeon, Delisa and
Miller, 1980) particularly where the therapist is working with children who have cancer and their families. This is due, in part, to the
small number of therapists working in oncology and paediatrics.
This number is, however, increasing, reflecting the increasing awareness of how occupational therapy is able to meet some of the
complex needs of these client groups.

In recent years, changes in health care delivery and in society's
view of children have been reflected in the changing nature of paediatric occupational therapy. Clancy and Clark (1990) suggest these
changes in service are not only exciting but require careful evaluation:

> New areas of Occupational Therapy practice with children have
> opened up . . . Practice is both exciting and experimental and we have
> reached a point of needing carefully constructed evaluation studies . . .
> for the ultimate benefit of the client – the child and his family.

The occupational therapist working with children with cancer is
faced with unique professional challenges in that the children
present with a wide divergence of motor, emotional, cognitive,
sensory-integrative and social skills. The intervention offered by the
therapist needs to maintain and enhance these functions as they
relate to everyday activities:

> The outcome of Occupational Therapy Service delivery is always
> determined by the child's mastery of tasks and relationships necessary
> to actively engage in play, self maintenance, school and prevocational
> activities. (Llorens, 1976.)

Mehls (1982) describes the role of the occupational therapist in adolescent oncology:

> The Occupational Therapist working with adolescents who have malignant disease, seeks ways to help these young people maintain their physical, emotional, and social functioning in the face of a life-threatening disease.

This could also be said to be the role of the occupational therapist working with children who have cancer. Each child has to be viewed as a unique individual within his or her own particular family and social environment. In addition to the usual developmental and life changes faced in childhood, young people with cancer also have to come to terms with their health status, with having to spend time in hospital, and with interruptions to the whole family way of life. Occupational therapists, educated in physical and psychiatric medicine and human development, are in the unique position of having skills which enable them to deal with the complexity of issues arising from disease treatment, hospitalization and the impact of cancer on family dynamics.

Knowledge and skills are used in a practical way, mainly through the use of change-enhancing activities which are guided by the therapist to produce a response. Activities must be attractive to the child and must encourage the child's participation whilst meeting the therapeutic aims of the therapist in promoting change in the child's abilities.

Pratt (1989) writes:

> It is the mandate of Occupational Therapists to provide services that support the child's achievement of health through engagement in purposeful activities. Inherent in this mandate is a second: that Occupational Therapy Services must be relevant to the time, cultures, and environments that are meaningful to the child. Accordingly service programmes must be designed and carried out that use goal-directed, meaningful, and age-appropriate activities to influence the quality of human development and life adaptation.

Occupational therapists do not work with children in a vacuum, as individual children present with unique family, social and environmental backgrounds. Parents, in particular, are of paramount importance to the therapist and it is necessary to include them in any service planning or delivery.

Irrespective of the nature or severity of the child's disease, it is important to work alongside the child and the child's family. The family needs to be involved at all stages of intervention and should be informed of progress and any programme changes. The occupational therapist's professional experience and expertise is based upon education, and knowledge of disease, family dynamics and child development, whereas parents' expertise is based upon their experience with their particular child and family. Chesler (1992) has suggested that both kinds of knowledge (professional and parental) are crucial for treatment to succeed.

The therapist should express her recognition of the value of family involvement, encouraging interaction with family members and not isolating the child from the family. It is important to remember that any siblings in the family will also be affected by the sick child's illness and are likely to be trying to cope with their life situation with the absence of a brother or sister and with reduced parental availability.

Working with the dying child

At one time the death of a child was much more common than it is today and many families had to learn to accept the loss. Nowadays our own life experiences and belief in the ability of medicine to provide a cure may leave us less prepared for dealing with the death of a child and such a loss greatly affects not only the child's family and friends but also staff working with the child.

Much has been written regarding the child's perceptions of death (Bluebond-Langner, 1978; Kane, 1979; and Koocher, 1973) with researchers being strongly influenced by a Piagetian framework. Kubler-Ross (1974) has written on emotional reactions to death, and Bluebond-Langner (1978) describes the child's acquisition of information about the disease in terms of the following stages:

1. 'It' is a serious illness.
2. Names of drugs and side effects.
3. Purposes of treatments and procedures.
4. Disease as a series of relapses and remissions.
5. Disease as a series of relapses and remissions (death).

Bluebond-Langner states that although none of these stages is 'iron-clad', in general, children assimilated a significant amount of disease-related information before progressing to the next stage.

Bluebond-Langner's research found that acquisition of information and personal experience produced changes in the way in which children viewed themselves. She described the development of the seriously ill child's awareness of his or her situation as follows:

1. Well.
2. Seriously ill.
3. Seriously ill and will get better.
4. Always ill and will get better.
5. Always ill and will never get better.
6. Dying (terminally ill).

An understanding of these issues enables the therapist to design a programme that is sympathetic, which demonstrates awareness of the child's view of himself or herself, and which is developmentally appropriate.

As in other areas of occupational therapy, the therapist works with the dying child (or with the child on palliative care) with the aim of encouraging optimum independence and improving quality of life wherever possible. Picard and Magno (1982), reviewing hospice care, said:

> The presence of an Occupational Therapist in the hospice array of services points to a continued meaning of life, even if that life is measured in days.

Tigges and Sherman (1983) demonstrated how quality of life was improved by enhancing skill areas important to the patient:

> The Occupational Therapist must concentrate on making the most of the patient's capacity and independence in self-care, work and play within the constraints of their physical limitations.

In general, intervention requires a 'one day at a time' approach with the therapist taking care to really listen to the child and family in order to find out what is important to them. Whitley *et al.* (1979) write that:

> Dying children and their families need to discuss sensitive and traumatic subjects, requiring the Occupational Therapist to be skilled and attuned to communication skills crucial to the therapeutic process.

The core skills of occupational therapists enable them to offer a service that complements those of other team members and at the same time to provide a well-defined input.

Daily living activities

The occupational therapist will encourage the child to maintain his or her self-care skills for as long as possible.

School

The occupational therapist provides equipment and advises on energy expenditure, encouraging and allowing the child to maintain some degree of participation in schooling where desirable.

Play/leisure

The occupational therapist will adapt favourite activities and introduce new ones to meet the child's changing abilities and needs. The therapist will also use activities to encourage expression of feelings.

Coping skills

The occupational therapist may introduce the child (and family) to techniques such as relaxation to promote coping.

Environment

Where the child or family are not able to do the things they want or need to be able to, the occupational therapist may arrange for adaptations to increase independence or ease child care.

An important goal of any occupational therapy intervention is for the therapist to convey the perception that the child (and family) do have some control over their situation.

To achieve this, the therapist must be aware of social roles within the family and must respect the way in which the family is dealing with the impending death. Contact from the therapist should be supportive, enabling family members to maintain and develop new roles as appropriate. 'Identities are linked to our social roles. To take away the roles is to take away the identities' (Bluebond-Langner, 1978).

Service delivery

Chapman and Chapman (1975) described a model of health care service that was based on the individual's right to a healthful, productive life. It categorizes different kinds of service as follows:

- Life-saving – directed towards prevention of imminent death.
- Life-sustaining – directed towards maintenance of health and the prevention of disability.
- Life-enhancing – directed towards maintenance, restoration and development of the individual's sense of well-being, social productivity and self-satisfaction.

Occupational therapy clearly participates in the life-sustaining and life-enhancing aspects of this model. The therapist is involved in aspects of life-enhancement where maintenance and restoration may not be possible. When children are dying, quality of life is equally important and intervention goals must be established in collaboration with the child and the family in a sensitive and realistic fashion.

Service delivery follows a logical sequence, starting with direct medical referral or a request made at a weekly paramedical team meeting. The therapist then introduces himself or herself to the child and family, explaining the role of the occupational therapist and what it has to offer both child and family. From here the therapist will assess and develop a specific programme for the child.

Assessment

Assessment is based on facts, clinical judgement and the perceived needs of the child and carers. Evaluation for occupational therapy intervention is usually an informal process and includes talking to the child and the child's carers to gain information on the child's health and well-being, his or her abilities, interests, and the social, home and school situation. Observation of the child in play, and social and routine activities of daily living indicate to the therapist whether more specific assessments are required.

The therapist will also seek information regarding the child's disease, health and treatment from medical notes and from members of the multidisciplinary team.

Specific standardized assessments which may be used by the occupational therapist include:

Developmental assessments

- the Schedule of Growing Skills
- Bayley Scales II
- First Step
- Miller Assessment for Pre-Schoolers (MAP)

Motor skills

- Movement Assessment Battery for Children (Movement ABC)
- Bruininks-Oseretsky Motor Development Scale

Sensory integrative functions. (These include awareness, discrimination and recognition of sensory stimuli from the environment and the use of this information to direct motor behaviour.)

- Test of Visual-Perceptual Skills (non-motor)
- Test of Visual-Motor Skills
- Frostig Developmental Test of Visual Perception

Cognitive tests

*   Goodenough-Harris Drawing Test

Following assessment, the therapist establishes the aims of intervention which are initially most commonly directed towards establishing a good working relationship with the child and family. It is essential that both the family and, especially, the child are confident in the therapist's skills as a clinician and are able to express hopes and concerns that will influence the therapeutic process and the child's stay in hospital. As the child becomes more confident, the therapist is able to develop his or her goals in working with the child. Lansing (1977) has recommended that therapists working with children should establish intervention goals that are related to the following:

*   The development and maintenance of functions and skills necessary for performance of the desired or required occupational activities.
*   Prevention of inadequate development, deterioration or loss of the functions necessary to engage in play, educational, prevocational and the various self-maintenance activities.
*   Remediation or rehabilitation of dysfunction that impairs acceptable performance of daily occupational activities.
*   Facilitation of the child's adaptive capacity to influence his or her own life and health status.
*   Collaboration, communication and co-operation on the planning and achievement of goals with the child and significant others in the child's life, including the family and other service providers.

Although intervention goals can be described in general terms, each child's programme is created specifically for that particular child, the child's needs and his or her unique family situation. Some examples of the therapist's intervention are now given to clarify the occupational therapy process applied to specific children.

Case studies

Case 1
Name: Suzanne

Age: 10 years

Diagnosis: Rhabdomyosarcoma

Social history: Lives with mother and father. Has older sister who lives away from home.

Relationship with family members: Has close relationship with parents and sister, appears to communicate well with family members.

Presenting problems/symptoms: General weakness, fearful of being in hospital and of treatment. Withdrawn.

Treatment: Chemotherapy, radiotherapy, surgery.

Is child aware of disease/diagnosis? Aware that disease is serious but not aware of diagnosis.

Initially Suzanne presented as being a scared girl who was unhappy about the treatment she was receiving and did not like her parents leaving her. She reported discomfort and was often sick or complained of nausea. The therapist together with Suzanne's family decided it was most important to achieve the following goals before proceeding further:

• Establish a good relationship with Suzanne and her family.
• Promote the concept that Suzanne had a large degree of control over any therapeutic intervention regarding the occupational therapy programme.
• Develop Suzanne's adaptive capacities to encourage a feeling of control.

Goals were achieved by spending time with Suzanne and her family to find out what she liked and disliked. The therapist was available daily and Suzanne was encouraged to decide if she wanted to see the therapist. She was given the choice of when she would like to see the therapist (within scheduling commitments) and what would be done during sessions. On occasion the therapist used some persuasion to encourage involvement in the programme but on the whole this was not necessary and Suzanne participated well.

The activities used were mainly creative as Suzanne particularly enjoyed making things and was able to express herself through this medium. The therapist also introduced breathing exercises and relaxation, encouraging Suzanne to practise these techniques, especially if she was concerned about receiving treatment or her parents having to leave her. It was also hoped that, by focusing on something constructive, Suzanne would be less inclined to think about her discomfort and nausea.

As Suzanne's treatment progressed, sickness became less of a problem and she was able to increase her physical activity. Goals of treatment were adapted to meet Suzanne's changing situation as follows:

- Increase stamina and mobility.
- Maintain level of independence in activities of daily living (ADL).
- Encourage participation in new activities to allow new avenues for self-expression.
- Encourage interaction where possible with other children on the ward.

Activities used included those already mentioned. Suzanne was encouraged to stand during sessions and, when her condition allowed, to attend the Occupational Therapy Department where it was possible to greatly increase her level of mobility and also to introduce more varied and challenging activities such as baking and clay modelling.

Suzanne's family was also encouraged to participate in her programme and the parents' group, which her mother has frequently attended.

Case 2

Name: Alison

Age: 7 years

Diagnosis: acute lymphoid leukaemia

Social history: Lives with parents, has one younger sister and one younger brother.

Relationship with family members: Good relationship with all members. Very close to mother who is the main carer while Alison is in hospital.

Presenting problems/symptoms: Extreme reduction in stamina following chemotherapy; weight loss in isolation.

Treatment: Chemotherapy.

Alison was first seen by the occupational therapist when she was under isolation conditions in a cubicle. She was lying on bed watching TV and said she felt tired and had not done very much since starting her treatment. Her mother was sleeping in the cubicle with Alison and caring for her. She was highly motivated in keeping Alison as active as possible but found it hard going. Both the mother and Alison responded eagerly to the therapist's offer of input.

Initial goals were:

- To develop a good relationship with Alison and her mother.
- To encourage participation in activities that require increasing levels of physical activity.
- To encourage self-expression through creative activities.

Alison responded well to the therapist's intervention; she was a creative child who enjoyed making things. The therapist graded activities, encouraging Alison to be as mobile as possible. Her standing tolerance increased quickly because she was often engrossed in what she was doing.

Sessions were often used by Alison's mother to catch up on shopping for special items of food to encourage Alison to eat, or to get away from the ward and have a cup of coffee.

As therapy was going so well, it was agreed with Alison, her mother and the ward staff that she would be able to attend the occupational therapy department where we would be able to used a wider variety of activities to promote increased function. It was also felt to be beneficial to take Alison away from the ward where she had been for some time and to a different environment.

Ongoing goals of the occupational therapy programme were to:

- increase stamina;
- increase gross motor activity in the upper and lower limbs;
- provide an opportunity to participate in purposeful activities, encouraging a greater degree of self-expression.

Alison continued to respond well in therapy and particularly enjoyed coming to the department where, on a number of occasions, she requested to do some baking. This activity was used by the therapist to meet all the above goals of the occupational therapy programme. As her physical health improved she was no longer required to stay in a protected environment. The therapist provided a wheelchair which allowed her mother to take Alison out of the hospital, only using the chair when she became too tired to walk.

The therapist no longer officially sees Alison as a patient but is pleased to see and hear of her progress when she attends clinic.

Case 3

Name: Fiona

Age: 10–11 years

Diagnosis: Brain stem glioma

Social history: Lives with her parents and one younger brother. Grandparents live nearby.

Relationship with family members: Good – particularly close to mother.

Presenting problems/symptoms: Increasing physical weakness and functional loss; tumour had not responded to treatment.

Treatment: Palliative care.

The therapist was initially asked to provide a wheelchair for Fiona prior to her going on holiday with her family. She was then not seen by the therapist (who was on maternity leave) until five months later by which time Fiona was wheelchair-dependent. Following discussion with mother it was decided that the most important area for the occupational therapist to focus on would be functional independence. Goals of intervention were as follows:

- reassess Fiona's wheelchair needs and provide a more suitable wheelchair to meet her changing physical abilities;
- assess her ADL abilities and assist Fiona and family in coping with increasing dependence;
- help her to maintain her level of independence for as long as possible.

Fiona's decreasing function made all ADL increasingly difficult and therefore it was more appropriate for the therapist to see her at home. A home visit also enabled the therapist to assess how the child was functioning in her normal environment. The first two visits were spent purely in assessing and providing the most appropriate wheelchair and supportive cushioning to meet Fiona's present physical needs while at the same time considering the inevitable physical decline that would take place. Psychologically, Fiona coped well with becoming wheelchair-dependent and her mother reported that she was keen to make the most of her increased ability to participate in activities outwith the family home facilitated by the wheelchair. This, however, was only in familiar situations or within the local community and Fiona was unhappy about any attention from people she did not know.

Other aspects of ADL were becoming more difficult and the community occupational therapist had already become involved to provide a stair hoist. A portable toilet was also used for a short time to save Fiona having to go upstairs to the toilet. Fiona herself did not appear too perturbed by her increasing dependence and the therapist associated this with the sensitive care provided by her family and, in particular, her mother.

Fiona was more concerned with other issues such as being able to continue doing activities which she enjoyed, so the therapist's next goals were to:

- enable Fiona to participate in activities that were meaningful and fun for her;
- introduce Fiona to new activities encouraging self-expression and encouraging use of remaining physical abilities;
- encourage Fiona's family to spend time with her in leisure/play activities.

This aspect of the occupational therapy programme was perhaps the most challenging to the therapist – having to devise new activities which were age-appropriate, interesting and could be adapted to Fiona's limited physical abilities. This was compounded by Fiona's great desire to express herself creatively and to participate in enjoyable activities with her family and some friends.

Simple board games were adapted using velcro and a communication system of eyebrow-raising and eye-blinking to enable Fiona to continue her participation. She was able to read her favourite magazines once they were positioned and taped to a book stand and household pegs were attached to individual pages to allow her to turn these independently.

The therapist found that adapting existing activities gave the family more confidence in doing things with Fiona and they became less worried that they would remind her of the things she was no longer able to do. It also gave a focus of attention for conversation, in which Fiona could participate, and promoted her participation in family activities.

Regular visits by the therapist also enabled Fiona's mother to have some time to herself knowing that the therapist would be able to see to any of Fiona's physical needs in her absence. Fiona's mother usually used the therapist's visits to catch up with things around the house but on occasions she would go out to have her hair done or go shopping. These outings were always planned in advance and usually the therapist and the Malcolm Sargent social worker did a joint visit so that in the event of Fiona becoming unwell, one person would be able to attend to her while the other could arrange assistance.

An important aspect of the therapist's input was to provide support for the family, especially Fiona's mother, who spent much of her day and night caring for the physical and emotional needs of her daughter. Over the year that the therapist spent visiting the family, the mother often took the opportunity to talk to the therapist about areas of concern and about how the family was coping with the situation. The therapist was also able to spend some time with Fiona's younger brother who was having increasing problems at school and becoming more uncooperative at home.

Following Fiona's death, the therapist attended the funeral and regularly telephoned the family. This has become less frequent as time has gone on and the last time contact was made was at a bereavement meeting. The family appear to be re-establishing itself in its new circumstances and has been able to enjoy a holiday abroad.

Adolescent groups

Youngsters may lose confidence because of their uncertainty about whether and how they will be accepted. Chesler and Barbarin (1987) reported that severe loss of opportunities for social interaction with peers may be experienced as a deprivation that multiplies other stresses of the illness. Positive interaction with peers may help the adolescent cope with the illness and renews the individual's adaptive capacities.

Perceived social support by peers is critical to adjustment among adolescent patients and Noll et al. (1993) suggested that teenage survivors appeared more socially isolated than were their peers. Other literature suggests that seriously ill youngsters tend to become more dependent on their parents, even if this is only a temporary phenomenon. For the adolescent this may involve a loss of newly gained independence, regressing to a prior dependent relationship.

A group run at an oncology centre was set up for adolescents. This came about because the occupational therapist working with a teenager identified the need for such a group. Discussion with Malcolm Sargent social workers followed and it was agreed that staff would approach adolescents between the ages of 13 and 16 years and invite them to attend a first meeting to play ten-pin bowling and discuss possible future events.

The group gives the opportunity for adolescents to experience popular activities in a supportive and non-threatening environment. Teenagers are encouraged to attend by themselves, or if they feel comfortable, to bring a friend or sibling. Some members of the group had also spent a period of five days at a Malcolm Sargent Holiday House where they were able to spend time getting to know one another and plan activities with some awareness of each others abilities. For most of the youngsters it was the first time they had spent the night away from home without their parents since developing their disease.

Aims of the group are as follows:

- encouraging development of positive coping skills;
- providing an opportunity for adolescents to regain or develop social skills;
- encouraging interaction with peers;
- promoting confidence by providing the opportunity to practise skills or develop new ones in a supportive atmosphere without parental involvement.

The parents of these youngsters have the opportunity of allowing their children to join their peers for a fun holiday, afternoon or evening in the knowledge that they are supervised by staff who are knowledgeable about the child's condition and, should there be a problem, will be able to seek appropriate help.

Parents' group

The family of the child with cancer also suffers and the parents may show greater adjustment difficulties than do the patients. Manne *et al.* (1993) found that 30% of parents assessed during the initial phase of their children's treatment showed clinically significant symptoms of depression. Maguire (1983) reported symptoms of depression and anxiety occurring in up to 50% of parents, although symptoms were usually mild to moderate and subsided after a number of weeks when the child began to respond to therapy.

Culling (1988) suggests that

> Removal of the family members from their home base and its social
> network may leave them feeling isolated and alone without the usual
> support network of friends and relatives.

Results of recent research indicate, however, that serious coping
problems are uncommon and that most parents develop positive
coping adjustment skills.

Many variables affect coping. Some of these may be fixed (such as
demographic characteristics, employment, social and other family
stresses), whereas others (such as level of knowledge and support) can
be modified. Monaco (1993) suggests that:

> Assistance in addressing family issues . . . is facilitated through the
> collaborative partnership among the family, Medical Care Team,
> parent self-help group and professional peer support networking.

It is well recognized, especially in the USA where much more information is documented, that parents can themselves provide support
and assistance in dealing with issues affecting families of children
with cancer. Families themselves understand what they need:

> We as parents for these children, are really a family, we must remember
> that even as one person's loss takes something from all of us, one
> person's victory gives hope and strength to us all . . . We will grieve for
> each other and cheer for each other, and most importantly, care for
> each other. (Tucker, 1990.)

A parents' group at an oncology centre in Scotland came into existence following comments by some of the mothers on the ward
expressing a frustration with sitting around all day and not being
able to do things for themselves. Everything they did was centred on
caring for their children and, consequently, they felt as though they
were neglecting other areas of life, attention to themselves often
coming at the bottom of the list of priorities.

Initially parents were invited to attend a meeting in a room close
to the ward, where refreshments were provided. Early sessions
focused on identifying the degree of enthusiasm for a group and
possible activities.

Response to the group is now mixed, with some parents attending
regularly and others not attending or just going when there is a topic
of specific interest. The degree of participation varies enormously
with some parents preferring to observe and others using the opportunity to express their feelings in some depth.

In addition to open discussion times, the following activities have
been arranged: keep fit sessions, relaxation sessions, Indian cookery,

aromatherapy and relaxation, ten-pin bowling, lunch outings and colour/style analysis. Activities reflect the interests of parents, and the facilities and time available to the therapist and parents.

No formal evaluation has yet taken place but parents' comments indicate that the group is a useful forum for meeting and getting to know other parents, especially for those who are new to the ward. It has also provided an interlude for parents during what can be a long day sitting by their child's bed.

Summary

In a small pilot study an independent practitioner found that, out of a group of 13 parents, 100% thought the occupational therapist's input had been helpful for their child and 4% said they themselves had benefited from the therapist's input. However, 7% said they would like changes to the service such as greater resources or an increase in the service offered.

Small study numbers make generalization of findings impossible, however, the study has highlighted the importance of evaluating the service offered. It may be comforting to know that all parents approached found therapy beneficial for their child, but the majority opinion that changes should be made in service delivery cannot be ignored.

Paediatric oncology is a new and highly specialized area of practice. Occupational therapy is able to assist the child and family meet the challenge of coping with cancer in a practical way, but for development to occur it is necessary for further evaluation studies to take place.

Action points

1. Describe the role of the occupational therapist in paediatric oncology in a unit that has never had this service before.
2. The unit/ward staff feel strongly that a family should not be provided with equipment – for example a wheelchair – to assist a fatigued child and equally fatigued parents. They feel that the child should be encouraged to walk instead. Discuss the occupational therapist's input, the decisions he or she would have to take, and where conflicts appear to have arisen.
3. A 17-year-old girl wishes to return home but requires a bannister rail, bath aids and chair-raisers if she is to be safely independent. How can the occupational therapist help the parents in persuading the rest of the family (three younger children) to accept this 'invasion' of their home?

References

Barnstorff P (1989) The dying child. In Pratt PN, Allen AS, Occupational Therapy for Children. St Louis: The CV Mosby Co.

Bluebond-Langner M (1979) The Private Worlds of Dying Children. Princeton, New Jersey: Princeton University Press.

Chapman JE, Chapman HH (1975) Behaviour and Health Care: a Humanistic Helping Process. St Louis: CV Mosby.

Chesler MA (1992) The child with cancer and the family. First Paediatric Oncology Social Workers' International Conference. University of York.

Chesler MA, Barbarin OA (1978) Childhood Cancer and the Family – Meeting the Challenge of Stress and Support. New York: Brunner/Mazel.

Clancy H, Clark MJ (1990) Occupational Therapy with Children. Edinburgh: Churchill Livingstone.

Cronin AF (1989) Children with emotional or behavioural disorders. In Pratt PN, Allen AS Occupational Therapy for Children. St Louis: CV Mosby .

Culling J (1988) The psychological problems of families of children with cancer. In Oakhill A, The Supportive Care of the Child with Cancer. London: Wright.

Dudgeon BJ, Delisa JA, Miller RM (1980) Head and neck cancer, a rehabilitation approach. American Journal of Occupational Therapy 34(4): 243–51.

Kane B (1979) Children's concepts of death. Journal of Genetic Psychology 134: 141–53.

Kielhoffner G, Barris R, Bauber D, Shoestock B, Walker L (1983) A comparison of play behaviour in non-hospitalized and hospitalized children. American Journal of Occupational Therapy 37: 305–12.

Koocher G (1979) Childhood death and cognitive development. Developmental Psychology 9: 369–75.

Kubler-Ross E (1973) On Death and Dying. London: Tavistock.

Lansing SG, Carlsen PN (1977) Occupational therapy. In Valletutti P, Christopolos F (Eds) Interdisciplinary Approaches to Human Service Delivery. Baltimore: University Park Press.

Llorens LA (1976) Application of a Developmental Theory for Health and Rehabilitation. Rockville, Maryland: American Occupational Therapy Association Inc.

Maguire P (1983) The Psychological Sequelae of Childhood Leukaemia: Recent Results in Cancer Research. Berlin: Springer-Verlag.

Manne SL, Bakeman R, Jacobsen P, Redd WH (1993) Children's coping during invasive medical procedures. Behaviour Therapy 24: 143–58.

Mehls J (1982) The role of the occupational therapist in adolescent oncology. In Tebbi CK, Major Topics in Paediatric and Adolescent Oncology. Boston, Massachussetts: GK Hall Medical Publishers.

Monaco GP (1993) Family issues. Cancer Supplement 71(10): 3370–6.

Nagy M (1948) The child's theories concerning death. Journal of Genetic Psychology 73: 3–27.

Noll RB, Bukowski WM, Davies WH, Koontz K, Kulkarni R (1993) Adjustment in the peer system of adolescents with cancer: A two year study. Journal of Paediatric Psychology 18: 351–64.

Peace G, O'Keefe C, Faulker A, Clark J (1992) Childhood cancer: psychosocial needs. Are they being met? Journal of Cancer Care 1: 3–13.

Pedretti LW (Ed) (1990) Occupational Therapy: Practice Skills for Physical Dysfunction. St Louis: CV Mosby.

Picard HB, Magno JB (1982) The role of occupational therapy in hospice care. American Journal of Occupational Therapy 36: 557–8.

Pratt PN, Allen AS (1989) Occupational Therapy for Children. St Louis, Baltimore: CV Mosby.

Reilly TP, Hasazi JE, Bond LA (1983) Children's conceptions of death and personal mortality. Journal of Paediatric Psychology 8: 21–31.

Robertson S (1978) Adolescents and dying. Medical Journal of Australia 1: 419–21.

Tigges KN, Sherman LM (1983) The treatment of the hospice patient: from occupational history to occupational role. American Journal of Occupational Therapy 37: 235–8.

Tucker K (1990) On guilt. Candlelighters Childhood Cancer Foundation. Journal 14(1): 5.

Weininger O (1979) Young children's concepts of dying and dead. Psychological Reports 44: 3955–4007.

Whitley SB, Branscomb BV, Moreno H (1979) Identification and management of psychosocial and environmental problems of children with cancer. American Journal of Occupational Therapy 33: 711–16.

Ziesler AA (1993) Art therapy – a meaningful part of cancer care. Journal of Cancer Care 2: 107–11.

Chapter 8
Occupational Therapy in Neuro-Oncology

Jill Cooper

Brain tumour

Lindsay *et al.* (1990) state that 'about 1% of all deaths are due to intracranial tumours'. As with other tumours, a brain tumour 'is an abnormal mass of tissue in which the cells grow and multiply without restraint, apparently unregulated by the mechanisms that control normal cells'. A brain tumour, once treated, may be cured, may be in remission for many years, or may recur. This cannot be predicted. Whether the tumour is benign or malignant, it still needs to be treated because it can be fatal if it is left.

The main distinguishing factor in brain tumours is that they arise in the skull. If the tumour grows and expands, it causes increased intracranial pressure within the inflexible bone casing of the skull. If it grows very slowly, some compensation for its pressure can occur, partly by displacement of cerebrospinal fluid and reduction in the venous spaces and partly by accommodation of the brain itself. Eventually, however, it can cope no longer: intracranial pressure increases and cerebral oedema often occurs.

A benign brain tumour

- can be successfully treated either by surgery and/or radiotherapy;
- the rate of growth is so slow that functional areas of the brain are not compromised;
- it can be treated and will not grow back for a very long time so the client lives a normal life span.

However, even if the tumour is benign, if it is in certain areas such as the spinal cord or brain stem it can cause severe dysfunction and be inaccessible for surgery.

Malignant brain tumours comprise cells that grow uncontrollably and may invade normal tissue. They may be curable and treatment is by surgery, radiotherapy and/or chemotherapy. These treatments aim to control growth of the tumour with the fewest possible side effects for as long as possible. Once treated, the cells may stop growing or multiplying which would mean that the brain tumour is in remission. Unfortunately, the tumour may recur later because it might not respond to surgery, radiotherapy and/or chemotherapy. It might grow back even when it had been thought that treatment had eradicated it. Alternatively, a new tumour might grow, its cells being undifferentiated from those of the original tumour.

The symptoms experienced by the client usually give a clear indication of its location in the brain. These may include headaches, paralysis, personality changes, behavioural disorders, failing vision, speech difficulties, epileptic fits, vomiting, papilloedema and sensory disorders – for example, difficulties with smell.

Diagnosis can be delayed because symptoms may be thought to be due to:

- cerebrovascular accident (CVA) – hemiplegia;
- epilepsy – seizures;
- brain metastases rather a primary brain tumour;
- head injury, particularly if the client had a fit caused by the tumour and injured his or her head;
- dementia.

Investigations will include:

- neurological examination;
- CT scan;
- MRI scan;
- X-ray;
- EEG.

Classifications

Brain tumours are classified according to the cells where they originate – for example, gliomas originate from glial cells. Souhami and Tobias (1995) list the following classifications of brain tumours:

- primary tumours: gliomas, pituitary tumours, meningiomas, pineal tumours, intracranial lymphoma, acoustic, chordoma, neuronal tumours;
- secondary tumours: common sites of origin being lung, breast and melanoma;
- gliomas account for 40% of brain tumours and are further classified into several groups as there are different kinds of glial cells (for example, astrocytoma, glioblastoma multiforme, ependymal tumours and oligodendrogliomas);
- astrocytomas are the commonest of gliomas. They are graded from I to IV, depending on their level of malignancy (I being least malignant). They can occur anywhere in the central nervous system, including the frontal, parietal and temporal lobes, the brain stem and the cerebellum of children. The slow-growing ones are called low-grade tumours (these are grade I and II tumours);
- glioblastoma multiforme are high-grade or grade III astrocytomas. The high-grade tumour may cause degeneration, necrosis, haemorrhage, infarction and local destruction.
- ependymal tumours account for 5% of adult gliomas and 10% of childhood ones; 85% are benign and are derived from ciliated lining of the central nervous system cavities;
- oligodendrogliomas account for 5% of all gliomas, the commonest age range being 40–60 years;
- pituitary tumours account for 10% of primary brain tumours. The pituitary gland helps control the body's hormones. These tumours are either non-secreting or secreting. They are usually benign but compress the gland, affecting normal pituitary function;
- meningiomas account for 10% of brain tumours, arising in the meninges.

Various other categories of brain tumours account for the other 40% of tumours and are described by Souhami and Tobias (1995).

Treatments

As much of the brain tumour is removed surgically as possible. Radiotherapy and/or chemotherapy are used to kill off cancer cells. Unfortunately, the blood-brain barrier works to keep harmful substances out of the brain and it may also keep chemotherapy out.

Steroids reduce inflammation. They do not kill cancer cells but they can improve quality of life by controlling the swelling of the brain, particularly before and after surgery. Anti-convulsants are often prescribed to avoid seizures caused either by disease or by treatment to the brain.

Radiotherapy can result in cognitive impairment which may be temporary and may occur at any stage of the treatment. It is thought to be caused by raised intracranial pressure, so regular evaluation is essential. There may also cerebral oedema which can exacerbate this. Cognitive impairment may also be seen in clients after surgery but before radiotherapy, among those who experience complications during treatment and may no longer be coping at home, and among those with tumour recurrence. In addition to impairment in processing information, recalling or retaining information, reasoning or making decisions, the client may be anxious, withdrawn, aggressive, confused or demanding and present with repetitive and unusual behaviour.

Cognitive impairment therefore has implications for occupational therapy, particularly with regard to safety when the client is unsupervised, the administration of medication, independence in daily living activities, resettlement into the community and psychosocial adjustment. It also affects the client's quality of life, ability to successfully return to employment, and compliance with treatment and rehabilitation regimes.

In order to manage these difficulties the occupational therapist should ensure that the environment contains the minimum of distractions so that the client can achieve optimum concentration. If appropriate, written material can supplement the treatment sessions and carers should be involved in treatment sessions whenever possible. A consistent approach should be used in close liaison with other staff, so there should be effective communication and planning within the multidisciplinary team. This will help the client to use his or her skills and abilities and will be useful in setting realistic goals together with the carers and the client.

Rehabilitation of the client who has cognitive impairment related to a brain tumour may involve functional and compensatory techniques. Different methods of performing daily living activities should be assessed so that clients can maintain their functional independence. They need to learn or recall skills to use in everyday situations as well as in rehabilitation or ward setting. This lessens the effect of the disability.

The functional approach is suited to perceptual problems as it involves repetitive practice, setting up a routine for clients and teaching them cognitive cues. Spatial and body scheme problems will still exist, however.

It may be possible to compensate for specific cognitive deficits to some extent by using remaining cognitive abilities, although one should not expect or aim for a return to normal functioning.

In order to achieve optimum level of functioning and safety and to plan management of the rehabilitation process and safe discharge home, clear rehabilitation goals should be set by the occupational therapist and carer, client or other staff. The client's environment may need to be adjusted depending on the level of impairment.

Visual impairment

Visual impairment may involve blurred vision, poor attention, hemi-anopia and headaches affecting eyesight.

In the UK, the Royal National Institute for the Blind have a range of products presented in brochures covering topics such as:

- daily living;
- clocks and watches;
- braille;
- mobility;
- learning and educational aids;
- leisure pursuits, games and puzzles.

The level of visual impairment and whether it is transient, permanent or likely to deteriorate will influence the occupational therapy intervention. If the prognosis is sufficiently long, the client may wish to learn Braille or be referred to specialist sources.

Equipment to assist people with visual impairments may include items that assist with poor vision as well as fine finger co-ordination, for example:

- egg-poaching rings; egg separators; an egg slicer/wedger;
- a kitchen timer;
- a liquid-level indicator, which clips to the side of the cup or other container; with sensors to indicate the level of fluid;
- oven gloves;
- double and expanding spatulas and tongs to give larger surface for handling foods;
- a can opener;

- large measuring cups and spoons with clear raised and indented markings;
- a chopping board with a raised edge;
- labour-saving devices – for example, a food processor or a microwave oven;
- a milk saver – a stainless steel disc which vibrates when the liquid is boiling;
- non-slip mats;
- audible clocks, thermometers, a rain alert (to alert the client to fetch washing in);
- a pill organizer.

Assessment of daily living activities can provide a baseline for management and demonstrates changes in the client's abilities before and after radiotherapy. The assessment needs to be simple and short as the client is unlikely to be able to tolerate a prolonged formal assessment. Reassessment may only prove that deterioration has taken place, which the client and occupational therapist probably knew anyway. Reinforcing the situation in this way is not appropriate. There is seldom any point in such an assessment for a high grade glioma with a short life expectancy and no potential for improvement.

Assessment can, however, detect subtle deficits and changes, which may possibly be difficult to observe consistently in interaction with the client but which can still produce gross effects on daily functioning. The occupational therapist may be able to suggest adaptive measures if such deficits are identified.

There should be an improvement in functioning from the middle of a radiotherapy course to the end of the course and beyond, and function tends to remain static and plateau two months after radiotherapy.

Hemiplegia

When a client presents with hemiplegia (paralysis in one side of the body), occupational therapy should aim to:

- counteract neglect of the hemiplegic side by working on that side;
- improve symmetry and poor balance by weight transfer and training for balance;
- facilitate normal movement patterns by inhibiting increased tone and avoidance of associated reactions;

- facilitate selective limb functioning and inhibit mass movements;
- encourage co-ordination, using bilateral activities or motor relearning activities.

Again, it must be emphasized that the prognosis may be so poor that return of function may not be achievable. This also applies to sensation loss, muscle weakness and poor balance and co-ordination. These symptoms may or may not respond to intervention.

Adaptive measures may include:

- providing equipment to assist daily living activities; this might include raised toilet seats, bath hoists and grabrails, and a perching stool;
- providing enlarged grips for cutlery and crockery;
- teaching rhythmic, repetitive movements to achieve tasks;
- teaching relaxation techniques to avoid frustration.

Information about the client's lifestyle can be gathered in a simple interview, covering the client's home, school/work situation and leisure interests.

Assessment

Assessment will examine physical factors (muscle strength, joint range of movement, muscle tone, sensation and pain), functional factors (self-care, mobility, perceptual abilities, domestic activities, work/school activities, leisure and recreational activities) psychological factors (insight into illness and response, motivation for rehabilitation and cognitive abilities) and social factors (the client's home situation, available support systems and carers' insight and ability).

The occupational therapist should consider the safety of the client and carer, the client's dignity and the need to involve the client as much as possible in decision making. If a client with advanced cancer, looking after two small children, is exhibiting signs of dementia, this should be referred to health professionals who will examine the causes for this deterioration. If the deterioration in behaviour is identified to be due to stress, the client could probably continue to care for the children with the support and supervision of social services, but when it is seen to be due to organic deterioration, it may be decided that it is not appropriate for two young children to be in the client's care for safety reasons (the client might leave gas on, etc.).

A clear and accurate diagnosis is, therefore, important in establishing the correct level of care for the client. This diagnosis should take place early on to ensure optimum planning for the client. Planning is necessary for issues related to housing, arranging power of attorney, and personal decisions (for example, concerning who should know the diagnosis).

The occupational therapist should provide emotional support and advice for the client (for example, reassurance that he or she is not 'going mad') and emotional support and advice for carers so that they can make sense of the changes that are taking place. The occupational therapist should also provide work plans for the client and carers, and take the opportunity to communicate where possible.

Clients may complain of unusual absent-mindedness, forgetting or mixing up words, memory lacunae (forgetting past events), difficulty in following books or films, and losing their thread in conversations or when carrying out elaborate procedures. They may also stare into space all day, experience significant changes in biorhythms (for example, sleeping during the day rather than the night), unexplained significant changes in eating or sexual habits, and difficulty with writing.

The occupational therapist should consider the clients' strengths as well as their deficits. They might, for example, still possess an intact knowledge base, good knowledge of certain subjects, intact social skills, social understanding, a sense of humour and relatively good language skills, particularly comprehension. Dysfunctions that are typically difficult to remedy include lack of motivation, agitation, short concentration span, difficulty proceeding towards goals and a tendency to be easily distracted.

Usual 'memory aids' may not work. For example, problems with keeping a diary as a memory jogger might be that the client does not bother to use it, does not remember to look at it, does not know what the day or week is and is not motivated to do the things that are supposed to be done on a particular day.

During verbal interaction, the occupational therapist can use prompts, for example 'I remember you said before . . .', '. . . before going on to do that, would you like to . . .', 'as I understand it then . . .', 'since you said that, I thought it might be helpful to . . .'

The occupational therapist should not be afraid to interrupt or move back to the main point, for example '. . . yes, shall we come back to that . . .' and should always avoid distractions.

Distractions should be reduced in daily living activities; the number of cues should be increased, for example to help the client in conversation using visual and verbal cues, and plans and routines should be thought through in detail. In assessment, observations should be made both when the client is subject to a lot of distractions as well as when there are few distractions, thus establishing whether distractions make the client unsafe.

The occupational therapist will need to consider the sorts of activities that the client will use to keep himself or herself occupied. It is important to consider those that may seem, at first, unlikely to be within the capabilities of the client as well as 'obvious' activities. 'Obvious' activities may include Trivial Pursuits, Monopoly, snooker, brass/string instruments, poetry reading/writing, verbal autobiography, verbal reminders, tile painting, computer games with immediate feedback, drama therapy, any activity that is accompanied. Unlikely activities may include bridge, Scrabble, table-tennis, keyboard instruments, novel writing and reading, preparing written autobiography, written reminders, quilt-making, computer games requiring strategy, play reading, any activity that is carried out alone. In order to build on success, the client's existing skills should be used and the carers should be encouraged to praise and acknowledge those activities the client manages.

The occupational therapist should provide the carer with a general explanation of the client's condition to enable him or her to understand what is taking place. The occupational therapist should assess the carer's ability and motivation to become involved in caring for the client, should encourage the carer to put aside some private time and should suggesting joint activities. Carers should not be overwhelmed with tasks that need to be carried out.

Special considerations should be given to cultural issues, bearing in mind factors discussed in Chapter 2.

Case study 1

Name: Mr P

Age: 50

Diagnosis: Grade III astrocytoma

Past medical history: Diagnosed two years ago and treated with radiotherapy for two months. No functional deficits identified at this stage. Presented two years later with poor short-term memory and left hemiparesis. Treated with stereotactic radiotherapy.

Social history: Married, no children. Employed as salesman. Very supportive wife who also works full-time.

Social support: No input as Mr P was functioning well prior to sudden deterioration.

Main presenting problems:

1. Left-sided inattention – i.e. requires prompting to pay attention to left side.
2. Poor balance and co-ordination. Mr P is a large man (approximately 18 stones).
3. Supervision of one carer for safety whilst carrying out activities of daily living.
4. Anxious about work.
5. Increased difficulty coping at home.

Occupational therapy aims:

1. To encourage awareness of left side.
2. To teach compensatory techniques for ADLs.
3. To liaise with physiotherapist on improving balance.
4. To work with wife and client regarding safety at home.
5. To reduce anxiety.

Occupational therapy intervention:
Physical and ADL assessments showed good right-sided muscle strength, dexterity, co-ordination and normal muscle tone. There was, however, gross left-sided sensory inattention causing poor balance and co-ordination with functional implications.

Functionally, Mr P was able to manage transfers slowly but independently although he was unable to get up from the floor or in and out of the bath. He walked unaided but unsteadily. He appeared to have dressing dyspraxia, particularly when orientating clothes and balancing to dress the lower half of the body.

Feeding was also affected by left-sided neglect. He was unable to hold cutlery in his left hand and food tipped off the plate.

He suffered from poor short-term memory, limited concentration and impaired judgement. It was difficult to assess his insight but it was clear that he could not understand why he could not go back to work.

A home assessment was carried out without him being present in order to discuss compensatory techniques with his wife. Adaptive equipment was provided to assist with eating and bathing and he practised with these in hospital. Options were discussed regarding organizing the home environment downstairs for safety. These were put to Mr P who expressed a preference to return upstairs but he agreed to being downstairs until he was able to manage stairs safely. This was a great relief to his wife who was the main carer. He was also persuaded to accept a wheelchair for longer spells out as, in addition to his poor balance, the disease and radiotherapy were very tiring.

Once he had accepted this, the occupational therapist was able to discuss smaller adaptations such as a rail by the WC and a bath for safer transfers, to which he agreed.

As he was unable to return to work, Mr P agreed to attend day care at the local hospice and, once he was familiar with the staff and environment at the hospice, he accepted Macmillan support. His wife found this particularly helpful.

He was discharged from hospital and gradual deterioration occurred. Mr P continued to verbally express his plans to get better and return to work. By gaining his trust, the team gradually helped him accept home care support as his wife was becoming too tired to help with his ever-increasing needs. Mr P, his wife and the team achieved his wish to be supported at home until his death.

Case study 2

Name: Mrs B

Age: 48

Diagnosis: Oligodendroglioma

Past medical history: Diagnosed one year ago, treated with surgery and radiotherapy successfully. Had epileptic fit six months ago, now on anti-convulsants and not allowed to drive.

Social history: Full-time manager in commercial firm, waiting for retirement on the grounds of ill health.

Social support: Husband (self-employed), and two teenage children, all very supportive. Husband is happy to drive her around but is restricted by his business; 17-year old daughter has just passed driving test so able to drive Mrs B.

Main presenting problems: Some degree of short-term memory impairment and frustration caused by this.

Occupational therapy aims:

1. To help Mrs B identify specific problems
2. To work with her to help her create techniques to compensate for her problems.
3. To teach relaxation techniques to reduce frustration.

Occupational therapy intervention:
Mrs B was referred to occupational therapy by the clinical psychologist who found that she had poor short-term memory, although this actually presented minimal problems upon assessment. The occupational therapist was asked to advise on practical issues.

A course of four sessions was arranged in which the occupational therapist helped to cover the above aims.

A long discussion in the first session identified what Mrs. B saw as her main problems. She already wrote reminders, kept lists, marked the calendar in order to jog her memory. She had worked full-time, had her husband and two teenage children to look after, and so she was finding it difficult to adjust to the sudden lifestyle change as she was now off sick. It reduced her self-esteem because she had been so busy and capable. Because she actually looked well, she felt guilty that she was unable to return to full-time employment (she had been signed off by her GP). The doctor was anxious that the stress of the job might initiate further seizures and she was clearly too tired to cope. Part-time employment was not an option because she would probably try to do a full-time job in part-time hours. Moreover, she was awaiting retirement on grounds of ill health and this had to be finalized before she could undertake part-time work.

There was a long frank discussion about the disease, treatment and the effect of the illness on her family and friends. As treatment had stopped approximately a year earlier, she felt some of them had difficulty comprehending why she was still off sick. The occupational therapist reassured her that her brain tumour was a very serious illness, and that she had undergone brain surgery (which left no visible mark as hair had grown back) and radiotherapy. Certain parts of the brain would have been affected so it was likely that there would be an element of damage albeit minimal and, beyond her own coping strategies, the occupational therapist could not suggest any others. What the occupational therapist could do, however, was to help her accept the situation, identify strengths and build on these, as well as teaching relaxation techniques.

The following objectives were identified:

- Mrs B would accept the fact that she had a brain tumour.
- Mrs B would accept that her illness was very severe and not feel guilty or a fraud about not functioning at her previous level.
- Mrs B would accept that she has all the free time she used to wish for when working full-time and that she should take back control and choice in her life.
- She would timetable activities that she had to do at present.
- She would compare these with a timetable of what she wanted to do – work part-time once medical retirement had come through, and work in a local charity shop.
- She would prioritize these.
- She would learn relaxation techniques.

Over the course of the following three weeks, Mrs B was able to accept the reassurance and she looked as positively as possible at her leisure time. She still had moments when she worried that her cancer would recur, which was understandable, and this was discussed. The occupational therapist could not honestly reassure her that this would not happen but regular check-ups and a recent scan did not suggest any evidence of recurrence. Beyond that, the occupational therapist advised she should arrange her time constructively.

Relaxation techniques helped her experience the contrast between feeling relaxed and feeling tense, so when she found she was becoming agitated or stressed she could practise breathing techniques or other relaxation techniques to produce the feeling of relaxation and calmness.

Although the sessions finished, it was agreed that Mrs B could contact occupational therapy if further problems arose. She was discharged from occupational therapy and was able to continue with her life as productively as possible.

Case study 3

Name: Mr E

Age: 36

Diagnosis: Fronto-parietal oligodendroglioma

Treatment: Radiotherapy
Past medical history: A single episode of epilepsy one year ago. CT scan showed left fronto-parietal tumour. Burr-hole biopsy showed

low-grade tumour. CT scan nine months later showed disease progression.

Social history: Lives with wife in own house. They have two little boys, aged two and four years.

Employment: Architect, employed full-time, very sympathetic employer who allows him to work hours to suit him and have an assistant draughtsman.

Presenting problems and symptoms:

* Proprioceptive difficulties in right hand (dominant hand).
* Control over right-hand grip.
* Acceptance of limitations on functional independence.

No difficulties with shoulder or elbow range of movement. Functional implications of difficulties included slowing down at work and an inability to carry out technical drawings unaided. Although the employer was very understanding, Mr E had very high personal standards and found these limitations extremely frustrating.

Occupational therapy aims:

* To assess Mr E's functional independence.
* To provide appropriate equipment to help adapt grip.
* To set a realistic treatment programme over a set period of time.
* To facilitate Mr E's acceptance of his limitations and advise him and his wife about coping strategies.

Occupational therapy intervention:

A course of four treatment sessions, once a week, was agreed with Mr E, the first involving assessment of hand-function activities and a long discussion of the practical implications of the illness. The disease process was also discussed to establish his understanding of his condition. Mr and Mrs E had a clear idea of his diagnosis, and the consultant had explained the prognosis. It was hoped that radiotherapy would alleviate the presenting problems but it was likely that deterioration would occur over the next year or two.

The main difficulties were identified and the following equipment was provided:

- triangular plastic pengrips and a rubbazote (large foam grip) for sketching pencils;
- a moulded cutlery knife ('Caring cutlery') as Mr E's fingers slipped off of ordinary cutlery;
- a programme of finger co-ordination exercises related to maintaining a full range of movement in joints.

Mr E was also taught:

- energy conservation techniques;
- hand-function exercises, together with encouragement to use both hands as 'normally' as possible.

Cognitive function was not tested as Mr E showed no obvious dysfunction, and appeared to fully understand and accept his disease.

Mr E managed well physically in adapting to decreased function in his right hand and developed good coping mechanisms. He invested in an electronic hand-held memo/notebook so that he could type in reminders and did not have to write very often. He still found it difficult to compromise his standards and slow down and he showed a high level of frustration. He talked frankly about this and the occupational therapist did not deny his anger as it was evident he was not going to resolve this quickly. Mrs E expected him to be angry about his condition and all parties agreed that he was entitled to be angry and it was not impeding his treatment or preventing him from getting on with his life.

Hand function continued to improve following radiotherapy and items loaned from occupational therapy were returned. Mr E continued to have his assistant at work and had grown used to the electronic notebook so incorporated these aspects into his routine. He returned to work, has regular follow-up appointments with the consultant, and he and his wife have the occupational therapy contact number should further functional problems arise.

Summary

Occupational therapy has a clear role in the treatment of brain tumours, both in the acute and palliative stages. It may include techniques used in other areas of neurology but the occupational therapist must be aware of potential difficulties due to fluctuations in the clients' performance.

The occupational therapist should be aware that clients have the right not to resolve anger and frustration that they might feel at their condition. The aims and objectives of intervention should be sufficiently flexible to enable the occupational therapist to work with the client and the carers whether the client has come to terms with the diagnosis and the dysfunction or not.

Action points

1. Select a neuro-oncology case study and describe it from a multi-disciplinary perspective.
2. A client with an advanced brain tumour is returning home from hospital. What advice and information could the occupational therapist working in the oncology or palliative care unit give to other occupational therapy staff and care workers in the community to help them be as effective as possible?
3. Discuss the occupational therapy approaches used in treatment of a brain tumour client and the process of reviewing performance at different stages of treatment, which in this case is radiotherapy.

References

Angevine Jr JB, Cotman CW (1981) Principles of Neuroanatomy. Oxford: Oxford University Press.

Grieve J (1993) Neuropsychology for Occupational Therapists. Oxford: Blackwell Science.

Lindsay KW, Bone I, Callander R (1990) Neurology and Neurosurgery Illustrated. Edinburgh: Churchill Livingstone.

Souhami R, Tobias J (1995) Cancer and its Management. Oxford: Blackwell Science.

Chapter 9
Returning Home

Jill Cooper

Preferred versus actual place of death

The place of death will often be a compromise between the wishes of the client, carers and health care professionals depending on the client's needs and the facilities available to support them. Ford (1984) observes that 'most patients prefer to die at home yet most of those whose place of death could have been planned still died in general hospitals'. Thorpe (1993) raises the related point that, generally, most of the final year is spent at home but most people are admitted to hospital to die. There are, however, some patients who do not want to die at home.

Over 40% of carers are over retirement age and more than half are spouses. Caring involves emotional stress, which may be excessive although it can be rewarding. Adequate support is essential to ensure carers can manage to prevent crises from arising.

Charlton (1991) conducted a survey of the views of people attending general practitioners' surgeries in England and Scotland on the subject of death and dying. The results showed that 63% of patients 'would prefer to die at home'. This corresponds well with the results from a study at the Northwick Park Hospital in 1990, where 58% of terminally ill patients interviewed wished to die at home in their existing circumstances, rising to 67% if their circumstances became more favourable.

The occupational therapist can assist in supporting the client at home, either by assisting with anxiety management or through the rapid provision of equipment. The findings also showed that leaving loved ones and fear of the unknown were most frightening and suggested to the author that good communication and counselling were amongst the most important tasks of health care professionals in this area.

A small study into preferred versus actual place of death published by Dunlop (1989) discussed how

> It is not surprising that 53% of the patients who made a choice should wish to die at home; a finding which lends weight to the recommendation of Lunt *et al.* about the need to make the development of home care teams an important priority. Home care services which are aware of the techniques and strategies required to promote security and good patient/family care can facilitate an increase in the number of deaths at home, or in the time patients spend at home before final admission but this may be more stressful for the relatives.

Dunlop further discusses the needs of relatives in relation to sudden unexpected death, the greater likelihood of bereavement difficulties for carers in this instance, and other related issues surrounding place of death and reasons for delay in transfers to hospice beds. He concludes that the study

> suggests that a majority of patients will continue to die in hospital even when hospital support teams, hospice and home care services are available.

Kirkham (1994) suggests that when people say they want to die at home it is more likely they mean 'when my days come to an end, I hope that it is in such a way that I am able to be at home' rather than a dogmatic wish regardless of their quality of life and disease state. He writes that Hinton (1994)

> interviewed his patients at weekly intervals for the first 8 weeks of follow-up and found that in the last 2 or 3 weeks prior to death, almost half of the patients who had previously wanted to remain at home asked to be admitted to a hospice bed if there was one readily available.

This did not upset the families of these patients who viewed their relative dying in a hospice as complementing the home care they had previously requested and received.

Maccabee (1994) states that:

> Due to the constant need for inpatient care, few palliative care/hospice units are able to allocate beds for long-stay care. This can lead to clients needing to be transferred to nursing home beds if unable to return home . . . The hospice movement has been powerful in focusing on the needs of advanced cancer patients as these needs relate both to acute pain and symptom control, and continuing long-term care.

The National Council for Hospice and Specialist Palliative Care Services in its Definition of Standards indicates that hospices should provide many specialist staff including:

- medical and nursing staff;
- staff trained to meet the psychosocial needs of the client, family and carers (for example, social workers, psychologists and counsellors);
- physiotherapists registered with the Council for Professions Supplementary to Medicine;
- occupational therapists registered with the Council for Professions Supplementary to Medicine;
- suitably trained staff to deal with bereavement;
- staff to provide spiritual care.

Nursing homes cannot, therefore, simply claim to provide 'hospice care'. Transfer to nursing homes may not be satisfactory to clients or carers. Thorpe (1993) observes that dying people who remain at home need:

- adequate nursing care;
- a night-sitting service;
- good symptom control;
- confident and committed general practitioners;
- access to specialist palliative care;
- effective co-ordination of care;
- financial support;
- terminal care education.

He quotes Herd (1990) who

found that admission became necessary because of:

i)   stress on relatives
ii)   the impossibility of providing more nursing staff
iii)   the lack of night sitters
iv)   absence of equipment
v)   absence of carer at home
vi)   symptom control
vii)   investigations.

If occupational therapists are to assist in maintaining clients in their own homes, they need to be aware of their prognosis and the likely pattern of decline of the client's functional performance. As much advice as possible should be sought from the medical team, although the medical team may not be able to give a completely accurate time scale and set of symptoms.

Planning the return home

A successful return home can include planned periods of respite care to allow the carers a regular break – for example, the client might spend six weeks at home and one week in a hospice or hospital. Sometimes less frequent admissions may be all that is needed – perhaps every few months to enable the carer to have a holiday.

The aims and goals of rehabilitation will be affected by fluctuations in acute symptomatic problems and the occupational therapist should be prepared to withdraw towards the terminal stages as the client is more likely to require nursing input nearer death.

James (1994) proposed that health care professionals have three important roles in ensuring that community care works:

- to develop an explicit view of themselves as part of a holistic health process that extends beyond the hospital setting and that includes not only the client but also the client's carers and those services relevant to successful admission and discharge into the community;
- to recognize that more time must be spent if patients are to be given a more active role in making their own life decisions;
- to manage the interface not just with their clients but with the variety of agencies that make up the as yet fragmented tapestry of community care.

The process for discharge planning involves:

- identifying the client's treatment needs;
- identifying the client's discharge needs;
- the clinician refers the client to colleagues, who may include the occupational therapist, physiotherapist, dietitian, speech and language therapist, the chaplaincy, the social worker, the clinical nurse specialist and the medical team;
- in-depth assessment and treatment by the occupational therapist;
- implementing the discharge preparation;
- MDT communication;
- liaison with relevant individuals in the community, including the client, the client's family, the social services occupational thera-

pist, the district nurse, psychological support, the home-care manager, the community physiotherapist, the Macmillan nurse, the community dietitian and the home-care nurse;
- establishing a package of care to suit the individual's needs;
- negotiating the discharge date with the community and the client.

When these stages have been completed, the client returns home with support services and discharge summaries.

The British Department of Health Circular HC(89)5, the Department of the Environment Circular LAC(89)7 and the accompanying booklet *Discharge of Patients from Hospital* highlighted the multidisciplinary team's responsibilities for helping clients return and stay at home. The main themes were:

Establishing discharge procedures

- Discharge procedures should be agreed with all those involved in their implementation.
- All wards and departments (including accident and emergency departments) should agree up-to-date discharge procedures which should be issued to all concerned.
- Procedures should be monitored by district health authorities in collaboration with social services.

Creating effective arrangements

- The doctor responsible for the patient should agree to the discharge.
- Doctors should have agreed, and managers should be satisfied, that arrangements for home care are comprehensive, as far as is possible.
- One member of staff should hold responsibility for checking that 'all necessary action has been taken' prior to discharge.
- Information from those at the receiving end of discharge procedures should be incorporated into a review of discharge policies.
- Consultation should play an important role in the review of procedures although a range of other professionals will also have a part to play.
- Details of procedures should be circulated to 'GPs, the ambulance service, local authority social services and housing departments and any voluntary bodies who may provide help'.

The UK Patient's Charter (1991) states:

> Before you are discharged from hospital a decision should be made about any continuing health care or social needs you may have. Your hospital will agree arrangements for meeting those needs with agencies such as community nursing services and local authority social services departments before you are discharged. You, and with your agreement your carers, will be consulted and informed at all stages.

Bone *et al.* (1992) suggested that the process of discharge planning has four phases:

- comprehensive client assessment;
- development of the discharge plan;
- referrals for the provision of discharge services;
- follow-up/evaluation.

This omits the important phase of agreeing a date for discharge with the client, carer and multidisciplinary team. The date for discharge needs to be established as far in advance as possible to enable all the services to be ready. Often, in the later stages of the disease, the team has to act quickly before the client's condition deteriorates.

In order to assist the team in discharging the client home safely, a discharge policy should be agreed together with a discharge procedure and individual health care professional responsibilities. An example of a discharge policy, from Warren Pearl Marie Curie Centre (1994), is given below:

Discharge Policy

Aim:
To ensure the provision of adequate arrangements which enable patients for whom discharge is appropriate, to be safely discharged. In pursuit of this aim, discharge arrangements will be conducted efficiently and compassionately and will be organised in a manner that permits minimum disruption to the patient and ensures maximum continuity between the services and carers involved.

Objectives:
1. The decision to discharge will always be made in consultation with the patient and family/carers. The absolute right of a patient and/or family to demand discharge will always be respected.
2. Whenever possible, discharge will be planned well in advance and preparations will always commence with the admission process.
3. The discharge process will be multidisciplinary and will involve both the hospital/hospice and the community health care teams.

4. Continuity of care between the Centre and the Community Health Care Teams will be facilitated by effective communication.

5. Maximum use will be made of available resources in order to ensure that the home situation is suitably prepared for comfort and safety and that the carers are adequately prepared and supported.

6. Where there are major obstacles to be overcome, short-term discharge with the option of planned respite admission will be considered as a possible solution.

7. Ongoing specialist palliative community care will always be arranged via the hospital/hospice's home care team or the local Macmillan nurses.

8. The patient and family will understand that readmission to the centre will be facilitated should circumstances require it.

9. All information relating to discharge will be recorded in the patient's nursing and medical notes.

10. All communication with community services will be confirmed in writing to the appropriate health care professionals/personnel.

The Discharge Procedure

1. Representatives of each clinical discipline will attend the weekly multidisciplinary team meeting.

2. Every patient will be fully discussed and those suitable for discharge identified.

3. A member of the multidisciplinary team will be identified as the key worker to commence and co-ordinate the discharge procedure for each individual patient.

4. Where the discharge procedure is logistically complex, the key worker will arrange a case conference involving all parties, including the patient and family/carers.

5. The progress of the discharge arrangements for each patient will be monitored at the multidisciplinary team meetings.

6. Completed discharges will be evaluated at the following multidisciplinary team meeting and will thereafter be subject to the audit process.

Occupational Therapist Responsibilities

1. Early referral to the occupational therapist is essential in order to enable discharge to be planned to a safe environment.

2. Inpatients may receive regular treatment with continual assessment and feedback to the multidisciplinary team.

3. Where problems regarding home circumstances are evident, a home assessment may be carried out with the patient, staff member and community agencies.

4. Where necessary, equipment required will be supplied and delivered and pre-arranged support from the community agencies set up prior to the discharge date.

5.   Further home visits may be necessary to continue with treatment and/or to demonstrate the use of or to ensure the correct use of equipment.
6.   Suitable patients will be considered for referral to Day Care.

Each team member should have their responsibilities and roles clearly identified.

Rehabilitation is an ongoing process which should start when a problem has been identified and not when medical treatment has finished. The occupational therapist approaches the client's problems as they arise and assists in organizing the provision of equipment on a short- or long-term basis as appropriate. Clients may also need the occupational therapist to help with anxiety management and energy conservation as they may not be well enough to resume their previous lifestyle.

Stump (1994) explains that the occupational therapy programme

> has to take into consideration . . . possible fluctuations in health, as well as pain, fatigue, depression, loss of skills, body image and functional mobility.

Once discharged home, the client can be followed up, distance and facilities allowing, to re-evaluate and modify equipment and services. Depending on local facilities and arrangements, the occupational therapist may refer to other social services or primary care occupational therapy colleagues for continued care.

Thorpe (1993) states that:

> Terminal care is an important part of palliative care. Not everyone dying at home needs specialist palliative care, but access to such a service should be available to anyone who does . . . Comprehensive terminal care requires scrupulous planning and co-ordination.

Client and carer choice

Discharge planning and organization for helping clients return and remain well-supported in their own homes form a large part of the occupational therapist's role.

In order to enable and facilitate the client in staying in their own home, the client and carer need to play a key role in making decisions. This means:

- the client and carer should be motivated to take decisions;
- the occupational therapist should establish where and how the client and carer wish to be supported;

- resources should be available at local level;
- there should be emotional, spiritual and physical support.

Mark (1994) states:

> That carers should be integral to the discharge process is not just a part of good practice; a prospective study (Roudot-Thoraval *et al.* 1987) demonstrated that the opinion of the patient or family (or both) was the best measure for predicting transfer to long-term care after acute care.

Berquist and Jacket (1993) place emphasis on 'goal development' rather than 'goal imposition' and point out that clients are not motivated to pursue goals that do not have any meaning for them. When clients are actively involved in making decisions their compliance is likely to be greater.

Occupational therapy home assessments

The occupational therapist may decide that it is appropriate to assess the client in his or her own home prior to discharge from hospital. The occupational therapist might choose to visit the client's home or accommodation without the client to assess the environment. This might take place, for example, if it is envisaged that the client will be discharged home to die. The occupational therapist can assess the client in the hospital department and gain his or her permission to enter the home or arrange to meet the carer there.

If a pre-discharge home assessment is felt to be appropriate for the client and he or she is well enough to go, this visit can help in psychological adjustment. The client will not be discharged home on such a visit and will need to return to the hospital or hospice until supporting services can be arranged. This gives the client and the carers time to prepare mentally for the return home. Continued therapy during this period will help with transfers and mobility, as well as providing time to train carers in the use of equipment (such as hoists) and transfer techniques (in and out of bed or chair or car, on and off wheelchair or toilet).

If the client does attend the home assessment, the occupational therapist should be aware of the relevant standard specified by the College of Occupational Therapists, *Home Assessments with Hospital In-Patients*. This covers referrals, procedures/policies, safety and security, assessment and treatment, and staff awareness. It also provides a checklist. It is important that the multidisciplinary team understands the aims of the assessment and that it is not seen as:

- a trip out of hospital for the client;
- a cheap method of discharging the client;
- a pass or fail test. If the client does not manage safely, the occupational therapist identifies what is required to ensure safe discharge home, if appropriate.

Discharge home assessments are not appropriate because:

- the occupational therapist is not legally able to discharge the client – this is the medical practitioner's decision;
- if the client is well enough to be discharged, he or she does not require an assessment;
- if a home assessment is needed, there will be concerns about the client coping so he or she will need to return to the hospital until services and/or equipment are in place.

Home assessments are time-consuming and are thus an expensive resource. They are cost-effective because they enable the client to be safely discharged and they prevent readmission. This service should not be undertaken lightly or provided without careful planning, however. Thorough assessment, liaison and communication is essential prior, during and after the visit. Clear aims and objectives should be set to ensure that home assessments are not carried out needlessly. Recording the assessment also forms a large part of the occupational therapy process. Home visit reports are required in complex discharge cases, with copies being provided to all relevant parties.

The occupational therapy home assessment provides:

- an opportunity for the client and carers to meet the community support in the environment in which care will be given;
- an opportunity for the carers and, for example, the district nurse to meet the client again in a better condition. The client might have been in a poor state of health earlier and might now be improved following symptom control and treatment;
- an opportunity for the client to reach a goal in treatment and be able to realistically envisage a return home;
- an opportunity for the client and the occupational therapist to walk around the accommodation together, thus enabling and facilitating the client and preventing the carer from being over-protective.

If the assessment proves that it is not safe for the client to return home and there is not an acceptable level of support available there, the visit has still been an important aspect of the treatment programme. The visit gives the client the opportunity to say 'goodbye' to his home – an essential step in accepting his or her circumstances.

The home assessment should include the following areas:

- the environment;
- establishing who owns the property as any necessary adaptations to be carried out will require the landlord's permission;
- establishing the type of property involved, whether it is warden controlled and whether it has any special features or arrangements;
- establishing with whom the client lives, the support network and community agencies involved;
- establishing the client's attitude towards returning home, and the carer's attitude including acceptance of the independence or dependence of the client;
- establishing whether the client is ambulant, or wheelchair-dependent, or uses a walking aid, and whether there is space in the home environment for safe mobility with such items;
- establishing whether there is sufficient access within the home: the entrance, steps, the threshold, door widths, accessibility with walking aids or a wheelchair;
- establishing whether the client is aware of change of floor surfaces and the implications of this for moving around with walking aids or a wheelchair – potential hazards, particularly loose rugs and unsafe flooring, should also be noted;
- assessing the need for transfers (particularly regarding the bed, chair, toilet, bath and shower). As much as possible should be assessed whilst the client is in hospital and it is important to consider whether appropriate equipment can be fitted on the visit. This may involve a social services occupational therapist being present on the home assessment;
- assessing the space and layout of the home with respect to their suitability for functional activities and the client's abilities relating to energy levels and mobility. The client's abilities – for example, in managing stairs safely – need to be considered if living in one room or on the ground floor is to be the solution.

Particular attention should be given to the following issues during the home assessment:

- *Toileting.* How accessible is the existing WC? Is a commode required? If a commode is needed, who will empty it? If this is a problem, would a chemical commode be the solution?
- *Bed.* Is the client able to transfer in and out of bed? What level of help is required? Will the bed have to be adapted to assist the client in lifting legs in or out? The height of bed needs to be considered in relation to postural support – for example, if the client has lung problems it might be more appropriate for the client to sleep in a more upright position. Should alternatives to sleeping in bed, such as the use of a reclining chair, be implemented? The ability to get up, washed and dressed, and the level of help required for this also needs to be assessed.
- *Bath.* Is bathing necessary for medical reasons or would a strip wash be preferable for the client? This can be established during the assessment in hospital. Arrangements may need to be made for the provision of bathing aids.
- *Kitchen.* How safe is it? Is a perching stool required? A wide range of equipment and adaptations is available. Functional and psychological abilities need to be assessed relating to preparation of drinks and meals. Would Meals-on-Wheels be appropriate or acceptable, or freezer meals? Particular consideration should be given to the use of walking aids or a wheelchair in the kitchen.

Other considerations may include shopping, alarm systems, entry-phones, ramps and rails. Keys may be made available for community agencies involved.

The occupational therapist should produce a written report following the home assessment. This should contain an assessment of observations and objective recommendations. Findings should be reported to the multidisciplinary team so that they can make decisions and plans for discharge. Referral should be made to community occupational therapists to carry out appropriate adaptations to the client's return home, if appropriate. These referrals may include drawings and instructions for positioning of rails. All completed paperwork, home assessment reports and referral forms, drawings, and so forth should be sent to the agencies involved promptly, including the nursing services and social services. The occupational therapist may need to ensure that access to the property is arranged so that work can be carried out. If the hospital or hospice facilities allow, temporary items of equipment can be fitted during the assessment to avoid delaying discharge.

Weekend leave without planned home assessments needs to be considered on an individual basis as it may prove to be an appropriate way for the client to establish whether he or she can cope safely. It allows the client and the carers to take some control by being able to report back on their needs and to decide what level of support they require. Occupational therapists should not impose their own standards.

Returning home may mean different things to different clients:

- they may wish to return home to continue with their previous lifestyle, either with or without adaptations to assist them;
- they may wish to return home to die, so time will be short and compromises may be needed to ensure they can be supported there safely;
- they may have experience of having returned home unsuccessfully before because of a deterioration in their condition – here the focus should not be on failure but on having tried and having been able to say 'goodbye' to their home.

If clients die before they can be discharged home, this can be frustrating for the multidisciplinary team. The team will have worked hard at making arrangements for the discharge. It is important for team members to realize that the planning process gave the client the hope of returning home so it was not a waste of their time and energy.

Occupational therapy services at home

College of Occupational Therapists (1993) lists the services that could be provided by occupational therapists to clients at home as follows:

- Daily living activities: advice, assessment and training towards independence in dressing, bathing, toileting, mobility, cooking, and so forth.
- Equipment: the provision of equipment together with training in its use to encourage independence in activities of daily living.
- Social skills: this involves assessment, programme development and training aimed at helping the client develop his or her own self-confidence and ability to relate to other people.
- Relaxation therapy: techniques can be taught to clients either at home or in clinics to assist problems with stress, anxiety, tension, depression, agoraphobia, panic attacks.

- Domestic rehabilitation: specific programme devised for individuals, for example menus, safety, joint protection.
- Ensuring that there is adequate access and providing adaptations where appropriate. This can involve providing advice regarding the situation at home or at work.
- Carers: advice, support, running carer groups.
- Paediatrics: programmes for children with special needs.
- Counselling: this can cover a range of issues including bereavement, cot deaths, miscarriage.
- Providing support and/or groups to deal with issues such as tranquillizer withdrawal, drug misuse and smoking.

At a practical level, Johnson and Harker (1996) advise on loan facilities for equipment in the community. The main issues here are:

- safety and hygiene: cleaning and storage of equipment;
- documentation: inventory system, written instructions for use;
- protocols: condemning equipment, operational policy, infection control and COSHH procedures;
- training of staff;
- finance and resources to maintain the service.

Case studies

Case study 1

Name: Mr H

Age: 78

Diagnosis: Metastatic cancer of the prostate.

Medical history: Prostate cancer diagnosed 25 years ago, treated over the years with chemotherapy. Metastases diagnosed 25 years later. Pain and weakness in legs.

Social history: Lives alone on the seventh floor of a council flat, with lift. Very supportive female friend, herself aged 75, who lives next door.

Social support: Friend, Mrs Q, was shopping for Mr H prior to his admission to hospital and sat with him every afternoon and evening. The district nurse visited daily to ensure medical needs were met and home carers helped with self cares.

Main presenting problems:

- Extremely emaciated and weak, which affects all transfers.
- Socially dependent on one elderly female friend, the district nurse and home carers to be supported at home.
- At very high risk of developing pressure sores.
- Difficulty planning to get home due to decreased functional independence.

Occupational therapy aims:

- To protect him from developing pressure sores.
- To enable him to achieve optimum functional independence – albeit only very little.
- To liaise with other health care professionals to provide appropriate help to support him at home.

Occupational therapy intervention:
Personal ADL assessment identified the need to help Mr H get in and out bed and to wash all parts of body other than face and chest. He just about stood and swivelled to chair from bed. Once he regained his strength after having a wash, Mr. H walked with a zimmer frame to the WC but was exhausted when he returned to the chair.

Domestic ADL was not assessed as he found domestic work too tiring and his elderly neighbour sat with him every day, making him cups of tea and light meals.

Home assessment took place with Mr H (in a wheelchair), occupational therapist, elderly female friend and district nurse in attendance. It was obvious that the client, friend and district nurse were all very fond of each other. Mr H was helped to sit in his favourite armchair, actually very low, out of which he was unable to independently transfer.

The home assessment comprised a gentle discussion with his friend sitting next to him, holding his hand, and the district nurse clearly glad to see him back in his flat. Over a cup of tea and biscuits, which Mr H was barely able to hold, he sat back comfortably and happily in his chair while the district nurse and occupational therapist discussed the level of help that would be needed to support him at home with him and his friend. This was designed not to rely on Mrs Q's input because of her age and health and because she was waiting to attend hospital for investigations. The suggested package of care included the following:

- home care would attend three times a day to help him get up, washed and dressed, toilet him, feed him and provide light meals;
- the district nurse would attend daily to check general health, to ensure that medication was being taken, check pressure areas and provide a pressure prevention mattress and cushion;
- hospice home care would provide night sitters initially;
- Mrs Q would continue visiting for company but not to provide any physical support as she was unwell herself.

The occupational therapist filled out the appropriate paperwork to have the armchair raised or, if possible, to loan a riser/recliner chair if one was available. She also requested a perching stool from Social Services, to be placed by the sink to help carers wash Mr H, and a raised toilet seat. Bathing aids were not appropriate.

Mr H therefore played a passive role but the occupational therapist and district nurse did ask his permission about suggested strategies. He was happy to leave the decisions to others.

After returning to the hospital he was very tired but seemed content. Liaison took place to instigate necessary services and a discharge date was set as soon as possible as he was very ill and wished to return home.

Two days prior to the planned discharge date, Mr H developed a chest infection and deteriorated steadily. He died in hospital and so never returned home.

Mrs Q and the district nurse visited him prior to his death and the occupational therapist met them on the ward. It was agreed that death was a kind release for him and it was a relief that he had not had to suffer or struggle at home. Although Mrs Q would have liked him to have returned home, it was likely that it would have been worrying and distressing for her. Despite the time and effort put into the home assessment and consequent liaison and plans, the occupational therapist was satisfied that, as circumstances stood at the time, it was appropriate to plan for him to return home. The services had tried to achieve his wish to the best of their ability. Moreover, Mr H was able to see his flat, say his 'goodbyes' to it and was clearly content that he had resolved any unfinished business. All were satisfied that he had died in dignity and comfort.

Case study 2

Example of home assessment report:

Date:

Name: Mrs F

Address:

Tel. No.

D.o.B. 1932

Diagnosis: Metastatic adenocarcinoma of rectum, diagnosed five years ago. Recurrence one year ago treated by colostomy. Commenced 5FU chemotherapy one year ago. Did not respond well. Admitted to hospital one month ago where signs of left L5/S1 nerve root compression were identified. Treated with two weeks' radiotherapy to pelvis.

Home situation: lives in owner-occupied first-floor flat with husband, aged 67. No children or relatives nearby. Prior to admission she had support from the district nurse once a week to look after her colostomy bag.

Home assessment

Mrs F was visited by occupational therapist at home on [date], the day after she was discharged home from hospital to assess her safety and functional abilities in her own home. Ward assessment had been difficult due to her fatigue and unrealistic perceptions of what she would be able to do once she came home.

Accommodation

Access: no difficulties with one step at front or back door. Communal hallway for flats. One bannister on the left ascending the flight of 14 steps leading up to the flat. Mrs F unable to manage this so carried up by ambulance men. The accommodation was all on one level once inside the flat.

Mobility: Mrs F was able to walk very short distances with a walking frame and with a foot-splint worn on left foot. Mrs F has a tendency to be unsteady and needs supervision by her husband. The flat is small and the distances from room to room are short.

Personal activities of daily living: Mrs F managed a strip wash with some assistance from her husband. Has urinary catheter *in situ*. Bath has vertical rail secured to bathroom floor level with taps, and horizontal rail across the width of the bath attached to the wall and vertical rail at approximately 30" from the floor. Bath is 23" wide and therefore not suitable for a standard bathboard (usually 26–28" long). Mrs F was not assessed transferring in or out of the bath as suitable equipment to ensure her safety was not available.

Domestic activities of daily living: husband manages all chores.

Cognitive abilities: in contrast to the unrealistic expectations expressed by her in hospital, Mrs F appears to be comfortably settled at home and performs safely within her limitations so she appears to have more insight. This may be due to her being happy to be home and in a familiar environment.

Summary

Mrs F requires supervision at times for safety when walking. She requires assistance with personal care to wash and dress, but can manage to transfer on and off the WC, the bed and the chair. At present, Mr F wishes to undertake this care by himself and attend to all domestic tasks. They have declined social services support, but have accepted support from the district nurse and referral to Macmillan nurses.

Mrs F is to attend the outpatients clinic again on ... by which time she feels she will be able to negotiate stairs again. Transport is available and Mr and Mrs F have been encouraged to make use of this.

The occupational therapist will review Mrs F when she next attends clinic.

c.c. Occupational therapy notes
Medical notes
District nurse and GP

Summary

It is recognized that change does not occur overnight. Factors that can improve discharge planning are:

* recognition that plans should commence at admission and should not be left until after acute problems are addressed;

- effective communication with multidisciplinary team;
- establishing discharge procedures and adhering to these.

Occupational therapists working in palliative care understand that their clients are dying, and need to be aware of the cumulative effect this can have on themselves emotionally and physically. If the occupational therapist can assist the dying client and carer to be supported in the environment of their choice, this is a vital contribution to their care.

Action points

1. Select a case study from your clinical experience of a client returning home. Evaluate how the occupational therapy process fitted in with the discharge procedure.
2. A client in the oncology and palliative care setting is discharged home and is readmitted very quickly. Identify the possible reasons for readmission, whether medical or social. Did the occupational therapy intervention need to be re-evaluated for improved discharge planning?
3. Outline a treatment programme from a multidisciplinary perspective to prepare the client and carers for the return home.

References

Berquist T, Jacket M (1993) Awareness and goal setting with the traumatically brain injured. Brain Injuries 7: 275–82.

Bone LR, Fahey M, Klein L (1992) Impact of hospital discharge planning on meeting patient needs after returning home. Health Services Research 27(1): 155–75.

College of Occupational Therapists (UK) (1993) Occupational Therapy in Primary Care. London: College of Occupational Therapists.

College of Occupational Therapists (UK) (1996) Home Assessments with Hospital In-Patients. London: College of Occupational Therapists.

Department of the Environment (1989) Discharge of patients from hospital. In Marks L (Ed) Seamless Care or Patchwork Quilt? London: King's Fund Institute.

Department of Health (1991) The Patient's Charter. In Marks L (Ed) Seamless Care or Patchwork Quilt? London: King's Fund Institute.

Doyle D (1980) Domiciliary terminal care. Practitioner 224: 575–82.

Dunlop RJ (1989) Preferred versus actual place of death: a hospital palliative care support team experience. Palliative Medicine 89 3(3): 197–201.

Ford G (1984) Terminal care in the NHS. In Saunders C (Ed) The Management of Terminal Malignant Disease. London: Edward Arnold, 202–17.

Herd EB (1990) Terminal care in a semi-rural area. British Journal of General Practice 40: 248–51.

Hinton J (1994) Can home care maintain an acceptable quality of life for patients with terminal cancer and their relatives? Palliative Medicine 8: 183–96.

Hinton J (1994) Which patients with terminal cancer are admitted from home care? Palliative Medicine 8: 197–210.

James A (1994) Community care and the clinician. British Journal of Therapy and Rehabilitation 1(1): 39–42.

Johnson M, Harker M (1996) An overhaul of home loans. Nursing Times 92(1): 60–2.

Kirkham S (1994) Admissions and discharges (Editorial). Palliative Medicine 1994 8(3): 181–2.

Leedham K (1995) District nurses' views on the role of rehabilitation in palliative care. International Journal of Palliative Nursing 1(3): 141–4.

Maccabee J (1994) The effect of transfer from a palliative care unit to nursing homes – are patients' and relatives' needs met? Palliative Medicine 8(3): 211–14.

National Council for Hospice and Specialist Palliative Care Services (1995) Specialist Palliative Care: A Statement of Definitions. Occasional Paper 8.

Ransford J (1995) Realising the Potential – Occupational Therapy in the Community. London: College of Occupational Therapists.

Royal Marsden NHS Trust (1994) Purchasing and Providing Cancer Services: A Guide to Good Practice. London: Royal Marsden NHS Trust.

Social Services Inspectorate, Department of Health (UK) (1993) Occupational Therapy: the Community Contribution. London: HMSO.

Stump N (1994) Home assessment before discharge from a palliative care unit. European Journal of Palliative Care 1(2): 96–7.

Thorpe G (1993) Enabling more dying people to remain at home. British Medical Journal 307: 915–18.

Further reading

College of Occupational Therapists (UK) (1993) The Therapeutic Intervention by Occupational Therapists with Consumers in their Own Homes. London: College of Occupational Therapists.

Pedretti L (1996) Occupational Therapy Practice Skills for Physical Dysfunction. St Louis: CV Mosby. (See especially Chapter 26.)

Chapter 10
Occupational Therapy in Hospices and Day Care

Jo Bray

Historically, health care has followed a biomedical model, disease and the physical symptoms of disease being the focus of the treatment. Hospice care has followed a more client-centred approach, focusing on the bio-psycho-social, and latterly spiritual aspects of care.

Hospices can be traced to medieval times when, it is suggested, they were established along pilgrim routes where they welcomed travellers, pilgrims, orphans and the destitute, as well as the sick and dying. Doctors did not associate themselves with such instituti ns as it was thought unethical to treat a patient with a 'deadly disease'. After all, they had their reputations to consider.

The word 'hospice' was first used to describe the care given to the dying by Mme Jeanne Garnier in Lyons, France, in 1842. The Irish Sisters of Charity established Our Lady's Hospice in Dublin in 1879 and later St Joseph's Hospice in East London in 1905. At about the same time other religious centres established care for the sick and dying throughout the country in what were commonly known as 'homes for the dying'.

The Marie Curie Memorial Foundation was established in 1948 with the aim of providing care for cancer patients dying at home with support from Marie Curie community nurses. Later a series of homes, which are now recognized as palliative care centres, were opened by the Foundation.

Developments in the hospice movement in the 1950s coincided with other medical developments: the discovery of new psychotrophic drugs – the phenothiazines, antidepressants and the anxiolytics – as well as the development of synthetic steroid and non-steroidal anti-inflammatory drugs, and developments in chemotherapy and intensive care units.

The most significant development in the hospice movement came from the planning and establishment of the system of care at St Christopher's Hospice, which opened in 1967.

This was also a time when progress was being made in research into pain management, the needs of the dying, understanding of bereavement and family dynamics. The most famous advance occurred in the 1960s when Kubler-Ross began her work. She later published her book *On Death and Dying*, which had a major influence on the attitudes of professionals and the public. It supported the need for the development of hospice care.

The medical profession began to address the needs not merely of the patient but also the patient's family, the main objective being to enhance quality of life until death. This dramatically changed the focus of care. The message was:

> You matter because you are you, and you matter until the last moment of your life. We will do all we can, not only to help you die peacefully, but also to live until you die.

These words, together with the concept of 'total pain' – not just the physical experience but also the emotional, psychological, social and spiritual elements of pain – were built into St Christopher's outlook and subsequently into the ideology of the modern hospice movement (Saunders, 1993).

Hospices have continued to develop over recent years and have moved away from their early image as 'homes for the dying'. The principles of hospice care have extended out of the physical hospice building into the community and also into the acute setting. Care is directed towards maintaining quality of life for the patient and family, so enabling the patient to remain at home. The National Council for Hospice and Specialist Palliative Care Services (1995) have produced the following definition of hospice care:

> Hospice and Hospice Care refer to a philosophy of care rather than a specific building or service and may encompass a programme of care and array of skills deliverable in a wide range of settings. The modern hospice movement has considerable public and professional support for a widespread network of hospices (NHS and voluntary) which, increasingly, base their practice on researched knowledge. However, the range and quality of the service are not defined by the use of the term.

Palliative care has long been associated with the hospice movement; however, it too has continued to develop and was recognized in 1987 as a specialty of medicine in Great Britain. The World Health Organization (1990) has defined the care offered by the palliative care multi-disciplinary team as:

the active care of patients whose disease is not responsive to curative treatment, control of pain or other symptoms, and a psychological, social and spiritual problem is paramount. The goal of palliative care is achievement of the best quality of life for patients and their families. Many aspects of palliative care are also applicable earlier in the course of the illness or in conjunction with anti-cancer treatment . . .

It goes on to say:

> Palliative care affirms life and regards dying as a normal process, . . . [it] neither hastens nor postpones death, . . . provides relief from pain and other distressing symptoms, . . . integrates the psychological and spiritual aspect of care, . . . offers a support system to help patients live as actively as possible until death, . . . offers a support system to help the family copy during the patient's illness and in their own bereavement.

Traditionally, hospices and palliative care have been associated with the needs of cancer patients and families. However, this now extends to those with any progressive illness as they will undoubtedly benefit from the principles and management of palliative care. This applies to conditions such as multiple sclerosis, motor neurone disease, muscular dystrophy and other neurological conditions, chronic heart failure and, in more recent years, the challenge of HIV and AIDS.

Hospices or palliative care units in Britain are funded by the National Health Service, or large national or local charities receiving some assistance from the National Health Service. They vary in size, structure and service provision. Services range from inpatient care, day care, outpatient clinics (medical consultation, lymphoedema management), domiciliary support from any member of the multidisciplinary team and specialist nurse advisors (home care teams) and hospice-at-home teams. Centres offer some or all of these services. Care is provided by an extensive multidisciplinary team including doctors, nurses, social workers, physiotherapists, occupational therapists, chaplains, bereavement workers and volunteers. Occupational therapy complements the skill mix of the multidisciplinary team.

The philosophy of the profession encompasses the principles of palliative care as defined by the World Health Organization. However, the recognition and employment of occupational therapists throughout hospices and palliative care units is spasmodic and is subject to local variation.

The National Hospice Council's Statement of Definitions (National Hospice Council, 1995) advises that specialist services should have an occupational therapist, registered with the Council for Professions Supplementary to Medicine, available full-time, part-time or with regular sessions. This should encourage existing and developing palliative care services to incorporate occupational therapy into their multidisciplinary teams.

Occupational therapy is an emerging profession within hospices and palliative care units. Historically, the role has been associated with craft work, the occupational therapist often being employed on a sessional basis. This may still be true in some day-care units where there is limited understanding of the occupational therapist's role. However, occupational therapists who are employed in units or centres on a full-time basis with a job description that defines their contribution as equal members of the multidisciplinary team (accessing inpatients, day care patients and outpatients) have a very different job from early occupational therapists in hospices.

The general aim of an occupational therapist's role is to facilitate independence through a process of rehabilitation. 'Rehabilitate' does not mean 'to restore to a former condition and status' when applied to the therapy provided to and received by patients with a non-curable disease. Bateson (1990) suggests that the term 'recomposition of life' is more appropriate as the occupational therapy process helps to build the client's life to a manageable level.

Dietz (1981) suggests that the goal of rehabilitation for people with cancer is to improve their quality of life for maximum productivity with minimum dependency, regardless of life expectancy. He further states that the rehabilitation process for cancer patients can be defined in four stages, and a patient can move between any or all of these stages:

- *Preventative rehabilitation* – treatment in anticipation of potential disability to lessen severity.
- *Restorative rehabilitation* – to enable clients to return to their premorbid status without significant handicap.
- *Supportive rehabilitation* – to support clients through their decline, the disease being progressive but stabilized, so that they can remain as functional as possible, retaining an element of choice and control.
- *Palliative rehabilitation* – to assist in symptom control, the disease being progressive and in its advanced stages, the rehabilitation preventing complications, for example through positioning, pressure care and preventing contractures.

In identifying these four stages the therapist is provided with a realistic treatment approach to facilitate patient-centred goals.

Palliative care, therefore, including that provided for patients with malignant and non-malignant progressive illness, focuses on the supportive and palliative rehabilitation stages of the patient's disease process.

It is imperative that occupational therapists have a clear understanding of the rehabilitation process within this setting in order to facilitate a realistic treatment programme. It is essential that they recognize their own limitations as therapists and that they appreciate the effect of suffering repeated failures by setting unrealistic goals that are never achieved, and which may result in increasing stress levels and eventual 'burnout'.

The occupational therapy profession is based on a problem-solving approach and, as with any other health care professional, intervention is based on initial assessment, goal setting, implementing the treatment plan, re-evaluation and reassessment. Within palliative care, this is an ongoing cycle. There is a constant re-evaluation process as circumstances and objectives change repeatedly over a period of time. The treatment goals of yesterday may no longer be applicable today. Occupational therapists must, therefore, be flexible in their approach to planning and to treatment.

Treatment programmes will be tailored to the needs of each individual patient and will also consider the needs of the carer. It is important to achieve patients' goals before implementing the therapist's agenda. It is essential that all goals are realistic, that they are achievable and continually reassessed, and that they are flexible in keeping with the patient's changing condition.

It is essential that occupational therapists convey to the client that they have unpressured, quality time to give. They must have highly developed communication skills in order that the client communicates his or her own goals and not those of the therapist.

The framework for practice is based on Maslow's hierarchy of needs. Maslow (1943) proposed that motives are organized in a hierarchy in which motives at lower levels take precedence over those at higher levels. Thus, motives at lower levels must be at least partly satisfied before those above them can significantly influence an individual's behaviour. In a similar way, the therapist is aiming to enable the client to achieve physiological needs (food, water, oxygen), safety (nurturance, money), belongingness and love (acceptance, affection), self-esteem (respect) and ultimately self-actualization (maximizing one's potential).

The feature of occupational therapy that separates it from any other medical profession is that it is the study and management of purposeful activity to enhance quality of life.

As the role of occupational therapy continues to develop within the speciality of palliative care, so the need becomes greater for theory to underpin practice. Reed and Sanderson (1984) described a model of occupational therapy that is known as the *human occupations model* (see Figure 10.1). The occupational therapist identifies the unique processes, concepts, techniques, concerns and assumptions and ultimately the outcomes of occupational therapy. The focus is on 'wellness' but this is not based on a medical model. The assessment addresses the individual's 'occupations', 'occupations' here meaning any activity requiring the individual's time and energy and thus using skills that have a value (a learned behaviour or a belief in something, for example). These occupations are related to 'self-maintenance' (washing, dressing, looking after oneself), 'productivity' (making a productive contribution to life, either in the form of domestic activities or by earning a living) and leisure. The individual must be able to participate in assessment and treatment and must also have the necessary 'components' to carry out these occupations, these components being motor, sensory, cognitive, intrapersonal and interpersonal.

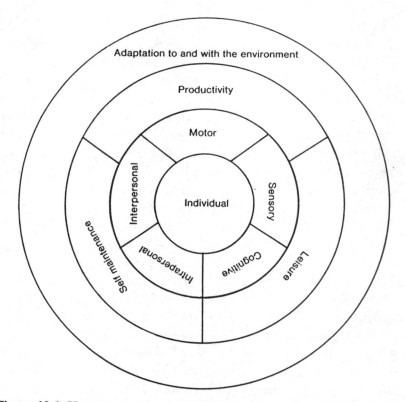

Figure 10.1: Human occupations model (an adaptation) reproduced by kind permission of Williams & Wilkins.

The terms in Figure 10.1 may be defined as follows:

- *Motor skills* – the level, quality and/or degree of range of motion, gross muscle strength, muscle tone, endurance, fine motor skills and functional use of these.
- *Sensory skills* – skills concerned with perceiving and differentiating external and internal stimuli.
- *Cognitive skills* – the level, quality and/or degree of comprehension, communication, concentration, problem-solving, time management, conceptualization, integration of learning, judgement and time/place/person orientation.
- *Intrapersonal skills* – the level, quality and/or degree of self-identity, self-concept and coping skills.
- *Interpersonal skills* – the level, quality and/or degree of dyadic and group interaction skills.
- *Self-maintenance occupations* – those activities or tasks that are carried out routinely to maintain the client's health and well-being in the environment such as dressing or eating.
- *Productivity occupations* – those activities or tasks which are carried out to enable clients to provide support to themselves, their families and society.
- *Leisure occupations* – those activities or tasks carried out for the enjoyment and renewal that the activity or task brings to the client. They may contribute to the promotion of health and well-being.

In using this model of occupational therapy, the occupational therapist takes a client-centred, problem-oriented approach, complementing the hospice philosophy in improving the individual's quality of life.

Motor skills

For many patients these skills are affected by muscle wastage or weakness which may be due to weight loss or weight gain. The result of this on the patient is loss of range of movement, a reduction in the ease of transfers or general mobility and fatigue. The early introduction and supply of equipment (for example, a bath board) may maintain clients' independence, thus giving a positive experience. As they decline, they may require additional support from a carer or professional. If equipment is supplied in the latter stages of decline, it is associated with that decline and viewed negatively.

Similar comments apply to the use and supply of wheelchairs. Clients may benefit from the supply of a wheelchair for long-distance outdoor use due to reduced energy levels and fatigue, however mobile they may be around their own homes and garden. Positive experiences and pleasurable memories all ease acceptance when the patient is limited further.

General advice can be given by the occupational therapist on energy conservation, how activities could be staged throughout the day, limiting stair climbing, and sitting while carrying out activities. Alternative techniques for carrying out activities can also be taught.

It is important to establish the clients' priorities, getting them to set the goals, to focus on the important activities, and to accept help from others in completing the less-important tasks.

Sensory skills

Patients experience many different degrees and varieties of pain, and often a patient's pain can be described as 'total pain', the focus of which may not be a physical sensation. It is important to recognize the width of the concept of pain and its influence over the occupations and activity when implementing occupational therapy assessment and treatment programmes. This may mean co-ordinating the timing of the treatment sessions prior to administering medication to facilitate optimal functioning.

Patients may have distorted sensation or a loss of sensation as a result of tumour growth on a nerve, or fibrosing of tissue, or they may have a medically induced loss of sensation for pain control. For these clients, advice and supply of equipment may be necessary to prevent accidental damage – for example, within the kitchen.

Loss of sensation decreases the patient's awareness of the development of pressure sores (the pain from such sores can have a dramatic effect on a person's well-being). The supply of appropriate cushions and mattresses is essential to the prevention of pressure sores. Occupational therapists have a wealth of knowledge on a wide range of pressure-relieving cushions.

Cognitive skills

Cognitive impairment may be a direct result of tumour growth within the brain or of secondaries. It may be as a result of side effects from medication or dramatic effects of fatigue. Those with direct tumour growth require a sound neurological approach to a treatment programme to be implemented by the occupational therapist.

All aspects of communication, comprehension, concentration and organizational skills need to be assessed by the occupational therapist as these are vital to the performance of occupations.

Intrapersonal skills

Poor self-image can drastically inhibit an individual's ability to cope with the 'occupations' and activities required in life. Feelings of anxiety and stress should be recognized and relaxation programmes should be taught to develop coping mechanisms to deal with such feelings in everyday life.

Patients whose 'occupational' performance is affected by their intrapersonal skills may need psychological support from trained professionals. In such situations the occupational therapist should refer the client to appropriate agencies. Goal-setting has the positive benefit of facilitating patients' involvement in, and subsequent control of, their lives.

Interpersonal skills

The disease often becomes the focus of patients' lives. They become disease-orientated; they lose control of their lives, they lose their roles and, in turn, they lose self-confidence, self-worth and self-respect. This is why patients should be encouraged to set goals – it gives them some control over their lives and increases their motivation and their positive feelings of self-worth. The use of a structured programme of activity within hospice day care can constructively use group work to enhance these positive feelings.

Having addressed the performance components or skills required by the individual, one then focuses on the occupational components, the activities in routine daily life.

Self-maintenance

This includes the skills necessary for personal activities of daily living: washing, bathing, dressing and toileting; and domestic activities: shopping, cooking, laundry, cleaning and general household duties.

The occupational therapist assesses the patient's abilities to carry out self-maintenance tasks. This assessment should not focus exclusively on performance outcomes/achievements but should also evaluate performance on those tasks that are of significance to the patient, and addressing how the client's goals in this field can be achieved. The occupational therapist will correct underlying problems, teach alternative methods or supply appropriate equipment in order to maintain independence. Those activities that are not of significance in helping the client achieve independence may be carried out by a carer or professional. Carers might also assist clients with their primary tasks. It is important that where possible the patient has the choice and thus can maintain control for as long as is feasible.

Productivity

It is important that clients feel productive throughout all stages of their decline. Many patients may have lost their employment, the role that was associated with this, their income, their role as a parent, husband, wife or family member, the focus of their lives being disease-led. Becoming a patient, an invalid, can give rise to feelings of passivity and dependency.

An occupational therapist can provide some structure or a new role to encourage productivity. This could range from advice on constructively filling free time following the loss of employment to helping the client exchange his or her family role from 'breadwinner' to 'housekeeper' or, if energy levels are severely limited, co-ordinating the shopping list for a home carer.

Leisure

Leisure covers the activities from which a patient gains pleasure. Everyone's psychological well-being requires that they gain pleasure or enjoyment for some part of every day. This is even more important for palliative care patients and, in assessing clients' occupational components, care must be taken to address this area, ensuring that energy levels and functional abilities still allow pleasurable experiences.

As clients decline their leisure goals are often small but they have immense significance to the client. It is important to recognize these and, where realistically possible, help the client to achieve them.

Day care

Sadly, very few day-care centres base their service provision on a sound theoretical framework or involve occupational therapy to its full potential. There is an immense area here to which occupational therapists can contribute, but it is one which is certainly not fully understood or utilized at present. A clear philosophy of care is necessary in order to achieve the aims and objectives of the service.

Day-care centres have grown in vast numbers since their initial establishment in 1978. There are now more day centres than inpatient palliative care units. Successive government reports have recommended that developments in specialist nursing services and day care should take priority over development of inpatient units. This strategy is in keeping with health care developments nationally promoting care in the community.

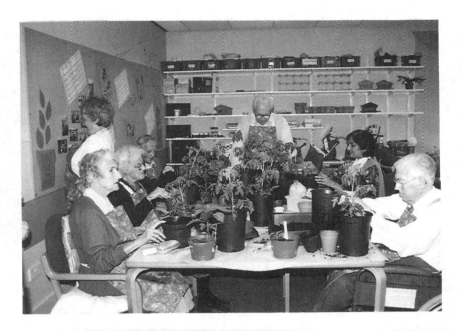

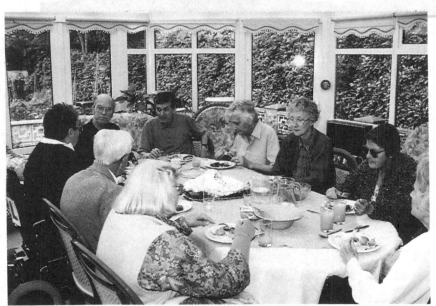

Figure 10.2: Patients attending day care, enjoying purposeful activity with specific aims and objectives as well as socializing with others.

		MONDAY	TUESDAY	WEDNESDAY	THURSDAY	FRIDAY
AM	Wk. 1:	Musical quiz	Sweet quiz	Red Cross: Hairdresser Aromatherapy Chiropody	Gardening quiz	
	Wk. 2:	Gardening quiz	Valentine's Day lovers' quiz	Newspaper group	Red Cross: Hairdresser Aromatherapy	Day care closed
	Wk. 3:	Faces you know quiz	Red Cross: Hairdresser	Outside speaker on Canada	Sweet quiz	
	Wk. 4:	Red Cross: Hairdresser Aromatherapy Chiropody	French theme day French quiz plus French lunch	Gardening quiz	Musical quiz	
LUNCH		LUNCH	LUNCH	LUNCH	LUNCH	
PM	Wk. 1:	Silk painting	Heart-shaped boxes	Art group/ Printing	'Thank you' cards Making cards	
	Wk. 2:	Painting terracotta pots	Making heart-shaped biscuits	Fabric baskets/ Birthday cards	Patchwork	
	Wk. 3:	Salt-dough animals	Concert	Painting terracotta pots	Salt-dough animals	
	Wk. 4:	*Papier-mâche* fish Painting salt-dough animals	Painting terracotta pots Making petit fours	Making biscuits/ Woodwork	Painting salt-dough animals/ Painting mugs	

Figure 10.3: 'Day-care timetable for the month of February' (Courtesy of the Warren Pearl Marie Curie Day Care Centre, Solihull.)

The future of palliative care services will probably be based in and around day-care units, with specialist teams of professionals supporting patients within their own homes. This will be cost-effective and will reach more patients than the present specialist services of inpatient units. Inpatient units presently cater for only approximately 6% of all deaths in the United Kingdom annually.

For occupational therapists to be recognized as part of the multi-disciplinary team, both within palliative care in hospices and in specialist centres and in the community, there is a great need to re-evaluate the occupational therapy curriculum. There is also a need for post-registration education and specialized courses.

The groups of clients undergoing day care tend to fall into two categories:

- some clients appear to be wrapped in cotton wool by their families or carers and so lose their roles and become introverted;
- some have no family but have carers attending so they take advantage of day care to communicate and may tend to dominate the conversation.

It is therefore important to select day-care members and to ensure that group dynamics are monitored.

Day care aims to:

- facilitate communication (discussions, newspaper groups, creative writing, reminiscences);
- focus on the calendar year (seasons, Christmas, springtime) as it could be the clients' last;
- provide group activity (collage for the main concourse, displays in clip frames in the corridor); past skills can be used and reintroduced in tabletop activities – for example, skills in horticulture or woodwork;
- provide activities that are achievable in one to two hours as the client may be unwell the following week;
- arrange social outings, concerts;
- encourage socialization, for example, at lunchtime to encourage appetite by making it a pleasant experience with minimal fuss and strain.

Statement of philosophy of day care at Warren Pearl Marie Curie Centre

'We recognize that all too often health care assigns sick and dying persons a role of passivity and dependency. We believe in valuing our patients' individuality and enabling the patient towards self-fulfilment and self-actualization.

'We believe that day care should provide patients with a stimulating and enjoyable day and that our care should be based on a sound therapeutic framework within which activities are selected for a specific purpose and graded to suit a patient's particular needs, thereby promoting confidence and self-worth.

'We believe our primary aim is to relieve isolation/loneliness by encouraging communication and identity within a peer group and secondly to provide respite for carers.'

'Criteria: This service is provided for patients with cancer who have evidence of metastatic disease or obvious deterioration from their primary disease.

'The Service: Mondays, Tuesday, Wednesdays and Thursdays at present, 10.00 a.m. to 3.00 p.m. Patients normally attend one day per week.

'Referral: Completion of the Warren Pearl Marie Curie referral form signed by a doctor.

'Transport: We have an excellent team of volunteer drivers providing a one-to-one service. Patients are collected at approximately 9.30 a.m. and return home by 3.30 p.m. If the need arises we can arrange ambulance transport for patients with mobility problems. However, this will be evaluated by one of the Day Care Teams [and will depend] on the patient's individual case.'

Case study

Name: Mrs R

Age: 67

Diagnosis: 13 years ago, cancer of the right breast. Mastectomy and 15 days' radiotherapy.

Two years ago presented with lymphoedema in the right arm

One year ago ulcerated right axilla

Right hand dominant

No functional use of the right arm, no active movement at all including shoulder. Referred to hospice and day care by the general practitioner.

Treatment: Pain control, lymphoedema bandaging for three weeks, now wearing compression sleeve and glove.

Social history: Widowed five years ago, lives alone, no family. Lives in a first-floor rented flat, access via one flight of 14 steps.

Social support: The district nurse visits twice a week to dress ulcerated area. Mrs R was very reluctant to accept help until she attended day care when home help was arranged to assist with shopping.

Presenting problems:

- Lack of use in dominant hand.
- Fatigue due to pain of heaviness of arm.
- Reluctance to accept outside help.

Occupational therapy aims to:

- Establish rapport with Mrs R to persuade her to accept help on her terms but not take away control.
- Establish areas of dysfunction.
- Set priorities for goals with Mrs R.
- Devise strategies to compensate for dysfunction.

Occupational therapy objectives:

- Mrs R will decide together with the occupational therapist the areas in which she will accept help in order to reduce fatigue.
- Occupational therapy assessment will be carried out in order to identify specific functional problems.
- The occupational therapist will prioritize these problems with Mrs R, ensuring she decides on the areas which are important to her.
- Mrs R and the occupational therapist will investigate techniques and equipment to facilitate independence.

Occupational therapy intervention:

Close liaison is always important with all clients, but particularly so with Mrs R who was so reluctant to accept help. This presented a difficulty for the occupational therapist and the team: they knew that they could assist her but as she declined help in certain areas they had to watch her struggle. However, this was her choice and had to be respected. Mrs R agreed to attend day care for a period of six weeks, on Mondays, during which time she was seen by the multidisciplinary team.

Dressing: The main issue here involved getting the compression sleeve on and off the lymphoedematous arm. A 'valet' frame was provided over which the sleeve could be stretched – this assisted with putting it on. If the home carers arrived early enough they were allowed to assist.

Mobility: Mrs R chose to wear a collar-and-cuff sling to support the weight of the arm. Although she had a bannister rail fitted to the right side of stairs ascending she declined the offer to have one fitted on the left. This resulted in her pulling herself up the stairs with her left arm stretched across in front of her, but descending the stairs was easy and comfortable.

Domestic ADL:

- Mrs R filled the kettle using a light plastic measuring jug with her left hand.
- She agreed to use small piece of non-slip matting to open jars and packets but declined a specifically designed jar opener.

- With regard to medication, she agreed to the district nurse setting out tablets in a Dosette box.
- Writing out the shopping list used up a lot of valuable time when the home help was there, so a portable manual typewriter was found which Mrs R could use to type the list before she arrived
- Mrs R declined a buttering board and preferred to place slice of bread on kitchen paper.
- She preferred to continue drying hand-washing over the bath on a clothes horse although alternatives were suggested.
- She refused to have the height of her electrical sockets raised for plugging in her radio.

The multidisciplinary team was able to assess her progress during the term of her day care attendance whilst also enabling her to take some control over her circumstances. Day care attendance also provided an opportunity for socialization and for participation in easily projects which increased Mrs. R's self-esteem considerably. In particular, she was able to make a small Christmas cake which she could offer to her district nurse and home help on their appointments. Mrs R declined to attend a local day centre despite having enjoyed the company at the hospice, but agreed to continue with regular assessments in day care.

Summary

As the field of palliative care evolves to concentrate on supporting clients in the community, the role of the occupational therapist in hospice and day care is expanding. The human occupations model helps occupational therapists to underpin their professional practice and can assist in defining their role more clearly in this setting. It focuses on the analysis of activities and the client's 'wellness', so the occupational therapist is able to address the individual's capabilities and to consider how to help with disabilities.

It is vital that clear therapeutic aims and objectives are set out for day care with criteria for attendance. These enable day care to provide an effective service both therapeutically and financially. The core skills of the occupational therapist are ideally suited for concentration on self-maintenance, productivity and leisure and for working with the multidisciplinary team in improving the client's quality of life.

Action points

1. A client is referred to day care and has never visited a hospice before. Outline an introductory package for new clients.
2. Discuss areas of research that are required into the role of the occupational therapist in palliative care, hospice or day care.
3. Examine the issues that occupational therapists face as a result of dealing all the time with clients who are very close to death. How do they complete their input when clients become terminally ill and require nursing care rather than rehabilitation input?

References

Bateson MC (1990) Composing a Life. New York: Plume.
Dietz JH (1981) Rehabilitation Oncology. New York: John Wiley.
Gibson A (1995) Creativity in the hospice – a celebration of achievement. Occupational Therapy News 3(5): 4–5.
National Council for Hospice and Specialist Palliative Care Services (1995) Specialist Palliative Care: A Statement of Definitions. Occasional Paper 8. London: NCHSPCS.
Reed K, Sanderson S (1988) Concepts of Occupational Therapy. 2nd edn. Baltimore: Williams & Wilkins.
Saunders C (1993) Foreword. In Doyle D, Hanks GWC, MacDonald N (Eds) Oxford Textbook of Palliative Medicine. Oxford: Oxford University Press.
World Health Organization (1990) Cancer Pain Relief and Palliative Care. Technical Report Series 804. Geneva: WHO.

Further reading

Fisher R, McDaid P (1996) Palliative Day Care. London: Edward Arnold.
National Council for Hospice and Specialist Palliative Care Services (1993) Needs Assessment for Hospice and Specialist Palliative Care Services: From Philosophy to Contracts. Occasional Paper 4. London: NCHSPCS.

Chapter 11
Models of Practice and Problem-Orientated Medical Records in Occupational Therapy

Jill Cooper

Models of practice can serve as concise explanations of the occupational therapy process, what it involves, and how and why it is carried out. If, for example, a client has died and the occupational therapist wishes to examine the value of his or her intervention, there is sound theory to underpin practice and reinforce the benefits of the occupational therapist's input.

Application of a model involves:

- defining core occupational therapy skills;
- selecting frames of reference and approaches;
- deciding on a model;
- using it in documentation.

Core skills

Before establishing a model or frame of reference, the occupational therapist needs to define what the core skills of occupational therapy are – what the expert knowledge at the heart of the profession is.

The College of Occupational Therapists (1992) describes the unique core skills of occupational therapy as:

- Use of purposeful activity and meaningful occupation as therapeutic tools in the promotion of health and well-being.

- Ability to enable people to explore, achieve and maintain balance in the daily living tasks and roles of personal and domestic care, leisure and productivity.
- Ability to assess the effect of, and then to manipulate, physical and psychosocial environments to maximize function and social integration.
- Ability to analyse, select and apply occupations as specific therapeutic media to treat people who are experiencing dysfunction in daily living tasks, interactions and occupational roles.
- Enabling people to maximize their physical, emotional, cognitive, social and functional potential.
- Anticipation and prevention of the effects of disability and dysfunction through education and therapeutic intervention in a functional context.
- Enabling people to achieve a meaningful lifestyle by the preparation for, or return to, work or the development of the quality use of time through leisure, education, training and opportunities for voluntary work.
- Provision of professional advocacy for people about matters such as access to premises and equal opportunities issues.
- Provision of practical advice and support for the families and carers of people with disabilities.
- Ability to change, adapt and modify practices according to the needs of people with disabilities and their environment.
- Ability to work in partnerships with others to facilitate the development of services for people with disabilities.
- The ability to influence social policy and legislation relating to impairment, disability, handicap and economic self-sufficiency.

Frames of reference

According to the College of Occupational Therapists (1992):

> The central values and beliefs of occupational therapy are that people with disabilities are valued as people with physical, emotional, intellectual, social and spiritual needs.

It continues:

> Occupational therapists use their core skills to enable them to empower people to make choices and to achieve a personally acceptable lifestyle, with the goal of maximising health and function.

This is the humanistic, client-centred approach to occupational therapy. It can be contrasted with the physiological frame of reference.

The physiological frame of reference is obviously based on physiology. It is concerned with maintaining the integrity and interactions of body systems, principally the musculo-skeletal, cardiovascular and neurological systems and the special senses.

One approach within this is the biomechanical approach. The biomechanical approach works on the assumption that:

- the application of a graded programme of exercise based on kinesiological principles will restore normal or near normal function.
- Biomechanical principles can be applied to the provision of equipment, orthoses or adaptive equipment to overcome residual disability.

Hagedorn (1993) says that the advantages of this are:

> Biomechanical techniques are well researched and can be shown to produce improvement in physical function. Because improving functional ability is the chief goal and results are relatively rapid, the patient can see positive benefits as treatment progresses and is motivated to continue. Residual disabilities can be overcome by equipment and orthoses.

To work purely within this approach risks the social, environment and psychological aspects of occupational therapy being ignored. Occupational therapists working in oncology and palliative care therefore use both the biomechanical approach and the humanistic client-centred approach, particularly using the latter with clients in the later stages of life. There is no point being prescriptive to those with life-threatening illnesses and the occupational therapist is there to help them achieve what they want within the limitations of our resources.

Humanists take a holistic view of the individual. This approach is particularly influenced by Maslow (self-actualization), Kelly (personal construct theory) and Rogers (person-centred counselling). This approach works on the assumptions that:

- The personal experience and consciousness of the individual is of paramount importance; no one should attempt to influence another's choices or interpretations of reality.
- The individual must be considered as a whole in the context of his or her physical and social environment.
- An individual has the right to personal choice (and all other human rights).

- The goal of occupational therapy is to enable the individual to be autonomous, authentic and self-actualizing (functioning as a free, self-directing, honest person whose life brings self-satisfaction and contains personal meaning).
- Individuals are capable of controlling events in their lives and should direct their own education or therapy as far as possible. An individual is innately capable of positive development.

It is a dynamic, holistic, flexible approach which can deal with psychological, developmental and physical dysfunction, and with deteriorating and terminal conditions. As a method of counselling or teaching the process is perceived by clients to be highly relevant; motivation is positive and results tend to be permanent.

Models

The core skills of occupational therapy, and the frames of reference, lead on to a model of occupational therapy that involves assessing and addressing the functional problems experienced by the client. Clients will all have functional problems – this is why they are referred to the occupational therapist.

Hagedorn (1993) observes that this *rehabilitation model of occupational therapy* assumes that:

> therapy should promote personal independence and should restore function to normal or near normal. Restoration of function can be achieved by graded practice of the damaged ability. Retraining should be carried out under realistic conditions with a view to the eventual resettlement location, social situation or work of the patient. Where residual disability persists, this may be compensated for by teaching the patient new skills or through the provision of aids, appliances, environmental adaptations or assistance from someone else.

Hagedorn continues:

> It provides a positive approach, aiming to improve necessary abilities, maximize existing function and compensate for deficits. It is highly practical, good at problem solving and a valuable, well understood, team approach.

The problem-solving model, which complements the rehabilitation model, works on the following assumptions:

- adequate data collection is essential for correct analysis of the problem;
- in any problem situation, there may be several applicable solutions – the occupational therapist should keep an open mind;

- problems should be tackled in an order of priority (but the order may be decided by the patient, or therapist, or pragmatically);
- the apparent problem may not be the real one: the apparent solution may not be the best one;
- interventions should be directed towards specific goals;
- progress should be monitored and action should be changed or the problem reassessed if results are ineffective.

The advantages of this problem-solving model are that it is highly pragmatic and flexible and avoids rigid thinking. It is suitable for all types of patients and can be applied to deteriorating or complex situations effectively. It promotes teamwork and provides measurable outcomes.

Outcomes

Reed (1984) gives the following as the desired outcomes of occupational therapy:

- Clients will be able to perform or will have performed those occupations that meet their needs.
- They will have performance skills that will enable them to perform self-maintenance, productivity and leisure occupations.
- They will have a balance of occupations such that actualization, autonomy and achievement are attained to a maximum degree.
- Clients will be able to adapt to the environment or cause the environment to adapt to them.
- Clients will be able to meet both deficiency needs and growth needs.
- Where the client is unable to perform skills independently, devices or equipment or other environmental adjustments will be used to compensate.

Problem-orientated medical records (POMR)

Many areas of clinical practice use problem-orientated medical records (POMR). This concept was introduced by Dr Lawrence Weed at the University of Vermont in 1969. The system is designed to promote a co-ordinated team approach to patient care with all disciplines treating identified problems. It takes different forms from one place to another but the principle behind the system remains the same.

This approach is particularly useful in occupational therapy because it looks at the patient, and both the aims and the process of treatment, not just at the disease.

Weed lists the benefits of POMR to the patient, therapist and profession as follows:

- it provides a standardized, recognized system of recording in medical and paramedical world;
- it is appropriate to all services – including psychiatry, geriatrics, and paediatrics.
- it can be used on computers;
- it provides evidence of the therapist's professional role and achievements for audit and research purposes;
- it provides a comprehensive, concise and fast method of recording without duplication;
- it facilitates easy retrieval of information;
- it facilitates improved communication and continuity of care;
- it facilitates improved use of the therapist's time;
- improved patient care.

The three main elements of POMR are:

- a database of personal information (such as name, address, date of birth, and so forth);
- problem lists;
- progress notes and discharge summaries.

The problem lists can comprise the following categories:

- *Motor* – mobility, co-ordination, muscle strength, muscle tone, stamina, range of movement, positioning.
- *Sensory* – auditory, visual, tactile, vestibular, proprioception.
- *Cognitive* – attention, communication, comprehension, conceptuality, judgement, memory retention, problem-solving, time organization management.
- *Intrapersonal* (psychological) – autonomy, coping, defence mechanisms, motivation, self-control, self-concept.
- *Interpersonal* (social) – group and individual interaction, social skills, values.

These allow the occupational therapist to establish whether there are difficulties coping in the following areas:

- Self-maintenance – for example, personal activities of daily living.
- Productivity – for example, homemaking, work.
- Leisure.

It may be argued that there should be a category for home circumstances. For example, if the client was unable to climb stairs, this could be due to motor, sensory or cognitive dysfunction. In practice, it is clear that it is an issue the occupational therapist should address. Occupational therapists working in oncology and palliative care might wish to use an adapted version with the following categories:

1. Mobility
2. Sensory
3. Perception
4. Personal 'activities of daily living' (PADL)
5. Domestic 'activities of daily living' (DADL)
6. Cognition
7. Psychological
8. Communication
9. Home circumstances
10. Work and leisure
11. Medical

The problem list is established after the patient has been assessed. The initial assessment/interview sheet identifies the main problem areas. The occupational therapist can expand on them in the treatment programme once they have been clearly categorized on the front sheet. Whenever an entry is made into the POMR, the corresponding problem number is inserted by the entry.

Documentation is carried out by using 'SOAP' notes. This stands for:

- Subjective
- Objective
- Analysis/assessment
- Plan

One of the letters S, O, A or P is entered alongside the entry. This enables the POMR to take the form of a comprehensive assessment that can be easily audited and used for reviewing and evaluating the patient's progress. It can also be used as a comprehensive report by other health care professionals, such as a social worker, care manager, physiotherapist, district nurse or Macmillan nurse. Other entries such as telephone calls and ward meetings can be simply written as seen in the examples below. The system can be used effectively by therapists working with multidisciplinary care plans or collaborative notes.

In order to reduce the ever increasing mountain of paperwork with which the occupational therapist is faced, the initial interview can be used as the main body of a function assessment for referral on to others.

Examples of POMRs

Example 1
Name: Mr C

Age: 81

Diagnosis: Cancer of the prostate with bony metastases, possibly spinal cord compression.

Past medical history: Diagnosed with prostate cancer three years ago, TURP (trans-urethral resection of prostate).

October two years ago, clot left leg, treated with Warfarin.

Long-term catheter *in situ,* changed every six to eight weeks.

Treatment: Ten fractions of radiotherapy from L4-S1.

Problem list:

1. Mobility (due to bony metastases, pain and weakness)

2. Sensory (due to numbness experienced in left leg)

4. Personal ADL (due to physical limitations previously listed)

5. Domestic ADL (as with no. 4)

9. Home circumstances (due to advanced years, elderly wife who has arthritis).

Date	Prob. No:	S O A P	OCCUPATIONAL THERAPY SERVICE INITIAL ASSESSMENT/INTERVIEW	Therapist's Initial
			Patient's Name: Mr C Hospital Number:	
June '96		O	SOCIAL SITUATION: Lives with wife, aged 79, history of osteoarthritis. ACCOMMODATION	
	9	O	Type: 2-bedroomed house Owned by: own/occupied Internal layout:	
			Downstairs rooms comprise kitchen, sitting room, hallway, dining room, outside toilet accessible by 1 step down from kitchen door.	
			Flight of 14 stairs with bannisters on both sides leads to:	
			Upstairs rooms comprising 2 bedrooms, bathroom, wc.	
			Community support: District Nurse 2 x weekly, home help 1 x weekly, good church support.	
			CURRENT FUNCTIONAL STATUS	
	1	O S	MOBILITY: Usually uses 1 stick, furniture-walks round house, but has been gradually off legs over 3-4 weeks prior to admission	
	1 2	O	STAIRS: Managing well with 2 rails but proprioception and safety affected by loss of sensation.	
	1	S	Transfers in/out left side of bed, reports difficulty with left leg, struggles at night.	
	1	O	Chair: no difficulties on/off armchair, 17" high, prior to hospital admission. Now dependent on 1 to transfer.	
	1 4	S	Toilet: prior to admission, no equipment required to help him transfer, managing emptying catheter bag with steady balance. Also has commode by bed.	
		O	Needs help of 1 to transfer.	
	1 4	S	Bath: Has shower over end of bath, has not yet been able to transfer in/out of bath for approx. a year	
	4	O	PERSONAL ADL: indwelling catheter. Continent of bowels, fell at home getting out of bed	
		S	on to commode.	
		O	Sits to wash, unable to stand unaided. Help of 1 required to dress, prefers to stay in night-clothes on ward.	
		S	DOMESTIC ADL: Wife manages with home help input.	

	O	COGNITION/COMMUNICATION: No difficulties.
1	P	Plan: Aim to achieve walking with 1 stick.
2	P	Aim to compensate for sensory loss.
4	P	Aim to achieve optimum functional independence.
5	P	Aim to achieve necessary level of help to support both.
9	P	Home assessment and aim to return home.
9	P	Multidisciplinary meeting Mr C to return to own home in approx. 2 weeks. Family meeting to be held to discuss discharge plans.
1	S	Client says that he has walked with a walking frame to/from bathroom and had a wash.
	O	Alert, sitting up in bed, lifting legs comfortably in/out bed.
4	A	Able to walk short distances consistently and attend to self-cares.
9	P	Home assessment planned.
		To practise bathboard transfers.
		Telephone call to wife to arrange date for assessment and meeting.
9	A	Home assessment. Full report written (not included for the purpose of this example), copies sent to all relevant agencies.
1	O	Successfully negotiated all steps and transfers.
4	S	Satisfied with progress and willing to accept bath aids and rail by WC.
		Discharged home successfully with services reinstated.
		Occupational therapy contact number provided to them should further problems arise.

Example 2

Name: Mrs D

Age: 58

Diagnosis: Breast cancer and recurrent cancer of the anal canal

Past medical history: Two years ago: Right total hip replacement for osteoarthritis one year ago, colostomy

Problem list:

1. Mobility

4. Personal ADL

5. Domestic ADL

7. Psychological

8. Communication

9. Home circumstances

Date	Prob. No:	S O A P	OCCUPATIONAL THERAPY SERVICE Patient's Name:Mrs D Hospital Number:	Therapist's Initial
30.4.96			Initial contact on ward. Initial interview sheet not completed as return home not likely at this stage.	
	4	S	Reports previously managing self-cares including washing, drying, toileting, feeding.	
		O	Sitting in chair, IV drip in right arm.	
		O	Appears low in mood, minimal interaction between client and occupational therapist.	
	4	P	For full ADL assessment by Occupational Therapist.	
		P	Occupational therapist to contact client's daughter regarding previous functional levels.	
2.5.96		S	Client too tired to assist in ADL assessment	
	1	O	Required to help move lying to sitting.	
	1	O	Leaned backwards and to the left.	
	4	A	Washing: independent sitting at the edge of the bed, washing face and chest when all items provided.	
	4	A	Dependent on 1 to wash and dry lower half of body.	
			Dressing: as above.	

	1	A	Chair transfers: needed 2 to move from bed to chair
	7		and needed verbal prompts to carry out shifting
	8	O	weight.
		P	Encourage independent sitting balance.
		P	Encourage independent self cares.
		P	Encourage interaction during treatment sessions.
3-10.5.96		O	Steady deterioration in function.
	9	P	Transfer to hospice for continuing care as prognosis now expected to be very short. Client and carers wish her to go to the hospice.

Example 3

Name: Master K

Age: 13

Diagnosis: Glioblastoma

Past medical history: Diagnosed 18 months ago, surgery followed by radiotherapy and chemotherapy. Currently on steroids resulting in peripheral neuropathy.

Problem list:

2. Sensory (due to steroid-induced peripheral neuropathy)

4. Personal ADL (due to steroid-induced peripheral neuropathy)

7. Psychological (decreased confidence at school due to recent illness)

10. Work and leisure (decreased confidence in play, schoolwork and sports due to recent illness)

Date	Prob. No:	S O A P	OCCUPATIONAL THERAPY SERVICE		Therapist's Initial
			Patient's Name: Master K	Hospital Number:	
1.2.96	2	S	Sensation in right hand 'feels as though I'm wearing a thick glove'.		
		O	Hand oedematous and concern that ligaments would stretch and deformity might occur.		

	4	A	Gross joint movements intact but fine joint move ments impeded by swelling.
	7 10	S	Felt self-conscious as hand enlarged, and frustrated as unable to join in with activities at school.
	2	O	Resting splint made of blue thermostatic lightweight material and matching velcro straps to ensure optimal joint positioning. Care of splint and instructions supplied.
4.2.96	2	O	Splint reviewed in occupational therapy department.
		S	Very pleased with it, comfortable and able to tolerate wearing it all evening.
		O	No reddened areas.
18.2.96	2	O	Splint continues to support hand, does not require adjustment.
		P	Continue wearing it as long as needed, review on next outpatient visit in two weeks.
	4	S	Is adapting well and able to manage one-handed self-cares to avoid damaging right hand until swelling is resolved.
	7	S	Feels happier now he has protection on the hand and school friends can see tangible splint. Also likes colour.
	7 10	O	Parents happy that play therapists and teachers on Paediatric Unit are able to help them as family and K's schoolwork is progressing well.
		P	Ongoing review as necessary.

Action points

1. Compare the models of practice and how they are best suited to working in the field of oncology and palliative care.
2. The occupational therapist is working in an acute hospital, treating clients with a diagnosis of cancer on an acute medical or surgical ward. Does the approach of this occupational therapist differ from that of one in a hospice setting and, if so, how? What are the aims and objectives of the treatment programmes of both?
3. Explore the advantages and disadvantages of having a joint note-recording system with other disciplines. Is this more efficient than occupational therapy POMRs?

References

College of Occupational Therapists (1992) Core Skills and a Conceptual Framework for Practice. London: College of Occupational Therapists.

Foster M (1992) The occupational therapy process. In Turner A (Ed) Occupational Therapy and Physical Dysfunction. Edinburgh: Churchill Livingstone.

Hagedorn R (1993) Occupational Therapy Foundations for Practice. Edinburgh: Churchill Livingstone.

Johnson S (1992) OT & Physical Dysfunction. Edinburgh: Churchill Livingstone.

Reed KL (1984) Models of Practice in Occupational Therapy. Baltimore: William & Wilkins.

Chapter 12
Occupational Therapy Standards and Auditing

Jill Cooper

The whole purpose of setting standards and auditing the service is to improve clinical care. The process involves investigating whether occupational therapists are doing what they say and presume that they are doing, how the service is carried out, whether or not it could be improved, and how to bring about any such improvement. Explicit criteria therefore need to be established for good practice.

If standard-setting and auditing are carried out simply and quickly, the process can be used in in-service teaching sessions and acted upon as part of normal working life. The results can also be used in reporting back on the service to management, as a tool to identify whether resources are adequate and to establish what changes are required and why.

Setting standards

The first step is to set standards against which the service can be measured. This is done before the system is audited.

Luthert and Robinson (1993) suggest that three factors that are essential to ensure the success of any quality assurance initiative are ownership, communication and leadership:

- *Ownership.* Staff applying the standards must agree to and understand the standards. If standards have been imposed in a 'top-down' manner, where management or external assessors who are removed from the daily running of the service implement the standards, staff will not be able to identify with them.

201

- *Communication*. There needs to be communication between senior levels of management responsible for quality of care and those actually carrying it out. This is so that the level of care defined is shared and endorsed throughout the organization.
- *Leadership*. This is required where change is necessary, particularly where there are resource or policy implications for the achievement of excellence. Those carrying out work need positive encouragement and full support from managers.

Advantages of setting standards

Sale (1990) discusses the advantages and disadvantages of standard setting. The advantages are:

- Standards can be written and monitored in clinical areas. They can be used to assess the level of service provided, identify deficiencies, communicate expectations and introduce new knowledge. They can also be written and monitored at the regional and district or organisational level.
- Standards reflect the therapist's own philosophy and values.
- Standards are dynamic and change in response to changes in practice resources and research findings.
- The very process of setting standards gives a group of professionals the chance to discuss and review their practice.
- Once standards have been set they can be incorporated into ward, department, unit and health authority targets.
- There is no need for a team of trained observers to monitor standards.

Disadvantages of setting standards are:

- Problems can arise from badly written or poorly articulated standards.
- Unfamiliarity with measurement techniques and the development of measurement tools may lead to unreliability.
- Setting standards is time-consuming.
- If standards are to be set effectively, they should be set by an individual who has experience of setting and measuring standards.
- Teaching staff how to set and monitor standards has resource implications.
- The activity of setting standards needs to be co-ordinated.

There are different ways of standard writing. One commonly used approach is the Donabedian model of structure, process and outcome. Donabedian suggested that standards of care and the way in which care is delivered must both be considered for a good quality service to be delivered. Standard writing can include the headings of structure, process and outcome as described below to explain what resources are needed, how they are utilized and what is hoped to be achieved. Higginson (1992) explains that '[s]tructure is the human, physical, and financial resources which provide health care. Its characteristics are stable and include the providers of care, of the tools and resources they have at their disposal, and the physical and organisational settings in which they work' (Donabedian, 1980).

'Process' refers to the activities that go on with and between the practitioners and patients. In simpler terms, Shaw (1980) described it as the use of resources. It includes measures of throughput and whether patients were assessed and treated according to agreed quality guidelines (Donabedian, 1980), such as treatment protocols. Guidelines are based on the values or ethics of the health profession or society (Donabedian, 1980).

Outcome is the result of the intervention. It is the change in a patient's current and future health status that can be attributed to antecedent health care. If a broad definition of health is used, such as 'the WHO (1947) definition of total physical, mental and social well-being, then improvements in social and psychological functioning are included.'

Wilson (1987) stated that a 'standard' was 'a definition of attainment' and that 'criteria' were 'the smallest of a hierarchy of definitions of performance'.

Luthert and Robinson (1993) suggest a framework combining aspects of the Donabedian and Wilson models (1987) and using the headings 'resources', 'professional practice' and 'outcome'. This can be seen in the Royal Marsden standards reproduced below.

The following are examples of standards of practice.

- Royal Marsden NHS Trust Occupational Therapy Standard of Care for Patients Undergoing Palliative Care
- HOPE Standards of Care
- Trent Core Standard for Palliative Care.

The Royal Marsden NHS Trust Standards of Care Project Occupational Therapy Standard of Care for Patients Undergoing Palliative Care

The following statement is taken from The Royal Marsden NHS Trust (1992). It illustrates the Luthert and Robinson framework outlined above.

1. Standard Statement

Patients receiving palliative care for their cancer will have access to a State Registered Occupational Therapist to improve and/or maintain independence and quality in all areas of life, to a level determined by the patient.

2. Rationale

Persons receiving palliative care may undergo different forms of symptom control depending on the nature and stage of the disease, problems may manifest themselves in a variety of physical, psychological, social and emotional ways. 'In response to the total health needs of the dying patient, the Occupational Therapist concentrates on enhancing occupational role performance in skill areas that are important to the patient' (Lloyd, 1989). Occupational Therapy can assist the patient and carers in identifying priorities and attainable short- and long-term goals and work towards these in order to improve and/or maintain independence and productivity in those areas of life.

3. Resources

i)   All patients will have access to a State Registered Occupational Therapist.

ii) The Occupational Therapist will have a knowledge of the philosophy of palliative care and the pathology of the disease processes as well as the medical treatment methods employed by the Royal Marsden NHS Trust and the potential side effects. The Occupational Therapist will have a knowledge of the principles of occupational therapy intervention and the support networks/resources available to the patient and family in the community.

iii) The Occupational Therapist will understand the treatment regimes of the Royal Marsden NHS Trust Occupational Therapy Department for the management of patients receiving palliative care.

iv) The Occupational Therapist will have skills in:

a) communication e.g. for effective liaison with other members of the multidisciplinary team and community services and to involve the patient's family/carers.

b) teaching – teaching family/carers/patient energy conservation.

c) practical techniques e.g. for safe use of equipment and for splinting.

d) analysing activities to establish patients'/carers' needs and appropriate occupational therapy intervention.

v) A referral system will be in operation.

vi) The Occupational Therapist will have access to on-going education programmes and support to ensure maintenance of the knowledge and skills base and to facilitate updated practice. The Group Head Occupational Therapist will organise departmental teaching sessions as appropriate.

vii) Other members of the multidisciplinary team will be available to act as a resource and source of referral to the patient, family and Occupational Therapist including the medical staff, community Occupational Therapist, physiotherapist, etc.

viii) Wherever possible the Occupational Therapist will liaise with the appropriate out-patient department clinics and be available to treat patients and give advice.

ix) The Occupational Therapist will have access to and the co-operation of the catering department for the provision of appropriate foodstuffs for patient assessment.

x) A range of 'Standards of Care' for specialist areas of occupational practice will be available to Occupational Therapy staff.

xi) Occupational Therapists will have access to medical information about all patients with occupational therapy needs.

xii) The Occupational Therapist will have access to a full range of adaptations and equipment for assessment and treatment purposes as well as validated and standardized occupational therapy tests to evaluate cognition, perception, sensation and functional activities.

xiii) The Occupational Therapist will have written information available to the patient and family including relevant instructions and safety precautions for any equipment loaned andwritten advice on how to cope with specific problems e.g. breathing and relaxation exercises.

xiv) Written information will be available to the Occupational Therapist e.g British Association of Occupational Therapists (BAOT) Standards, Policies and Proceedings including guidelines for home assessments, access to transport for these pre- and post-discharge, with or without the patient at the Occupational Therapist's professional discretion.

xv) The Occupational Therapist will have access to secretarial support.

xvi) The Occupational Therapy department will have access to an area that includes:-

a) a kitchen
b) a bathroom and toilet
c) a bedroom
d) a general treatment area
e) storage facilities
f) office accommodation and office equipment including telephone

NB The department will be wheelchair accessible and must comply with the Health and Safety standards at the Royal Marsden NHS Trust.

xvii) The Occupational Therapist will have available a documentation system to record professional practice. This record will be in the POMR (Problem Orientated Medical Record) format based on the Reed & Sanderson Model of Human Occupation.

4. Professional Practice

i) Upon referral, the Occupational Therapist makes an initial and on-going assessment of:
a) the patient's functional status including the level of self care, mobility, leisure activities and domestic activities of daily living, using recognized assessments and activity analysis skills.
b) the patient's physical status, e.g. pain level, lymphoedema, wound management and fungating lesions, energy tolerance which influences range of movement, mobility and safety.
c) the patient's psychological status including insight into illness, motivation and presence of anxiety.
d) social status including home situation and environment, and support agencies at home.

This assessment takes into consideration the patient's disease status, previous/current treatments and medical prognosis.

ii) The Occupational Therapist analyses the assessment and gives advice and/or agrees a plan of treatment with the patient and family to set initial mutual goals. These are re-evaluated as an on-going process.
iii) The Occupational Therapist implements a plan of treatment based on the needs identified in the assessment:

a) Where appropriate the Occupational Therapist assists patients to practice activities of daily living and teaches the patient and family alternative strategies/techniques which may include community support.
b) The Occupational Therapist advises the patient and family on energy conservation techniques and arranges for provision of necessary equipment to assist in this area.
c) The Occupational Therapist analyses joint dysfunction and provides static or active splints as necessary to improve/maintain joint positioning and function.
d) The Occupational Therapist advises on the appropriate equipment to assist carers and patients on its correct use e.g. wheelchairs, aids to independence, and pressure cushions.
e) The Occupational Therapist works with patient and carer to identify potential anxiety-provoking situations and how to deal with these by teaching relaxation techniques as appropriate to their needs.
f) The Occupational Therapist ensures that adequate support is arranged for both patient and carers via communication with appropriate agencies.

iv) The Occupational Therapist co-ordinates interventions with other members of the multidisciplinary team including medical staff, nursing staff and physiotherapists to ensure that the optimum level of function is attained and maintained.
v) The Occupational Therapist evaluates the effectiveness of treatment by continually re-assessing the patient and amends interventions as necessary.

vi) To ensure continuity of care is achieved on discharge the Occupational Therapist liaises with the community Occupational Therapist, the community liaison nurse, the social worker and/or social services, and the general practitioner as appropriate. The Occupational Therapist carries out a home assessment with the patient prior to discharge if this is appropriate.

vii) The Occupational Therapist documents all aspects of professional practice in the departmental records and where appropriate records Occupational Therapy treatment/intervention in the medical and/or nursing notes.

5. Outcomes

i) The documentation shows evidence that the patient achieved the goals determined by him/herself. If the patient's condition deteriorated, there is also evidence that the family's practical needs were met.

ii) The patient and family consider that the patient achieved the goals determined by him/herself. If the patient's condition deteriorated then the family felt their needs for practical support were met and that if the patient was discharged home that the arrangements and response of the Occupational Therapist were appropriate.

iii) The Occupational Therapist considers that he/she had access to the resources as listedand was able to follow the described professional practice. The Occupational Therapist also considers that the patient achieved the goals determined by him/herself.

iv) The patient and carer are satisfied with the care given.

HOPE Standards of Care

OCCUPATIONAL THERAPY SERVICE

TOPIC	Occupational therapy in palliative care
SUB-TOPIC	Optimal functional independence of patients and carers
STANDARD	Patients undergoing palliative care are seen within *hours of referral by a member of the OT department

STRUCTURE	PROCESS	OUTCOME
Referral procedure	The OT has access to the medical notes	Response to the referral takes place in *hours
Access to a qualified OT	The OT records the referral, the initial assessment, the outcome and recommendations	There is written evidence of the referral, assessment, identifying negotiated aims and objectives with patient/and carer.

OT departmental policies and procedures complying with BOAT guidelines		There is written evidence of a treatment programme, use of media, identifying the OT process
Health Authority/ Unit policies and procedures		

OCCUPATIONAL THERAPY SERVICE

TOPIC	Day care
SUB-TOPIC	Reassessment of day care patients/members
STANDARD	Patients are re-evaluated/re-assessed at three-monthly intervals

STRUCTURE	PROCESS	OUTCOME
Assessment is carried out by designated member of the day care team	Review date made with member of staff and patient	There is written evidence of next review date
An environment conducive to confidentiality is available	Pre-booking of available rooms is recorded	Patients are re-evaluated at three-monthly intervals
There is a policy for review of day care patients in operation	The member of staff records the initial and subsequent assessments, noting the outcome and recommendations	There is written evidence of the assessment
		There is written evidence of action taken to other referral agencies

OCCUPATIONAL THERAPY SERVICE

TOPIC	Communication
SUB-TOPIC	Patient communication
STANDARD	All patients are offered structure group work to facilitate communication and interaction

STRUCTURE	PROCESS	OUTCOME
Staff – minimum 2	1 A member of staff ensures that each patient is comfortable and ready to participate in the	All members of the group have communicated during the activity
Warm room – minimum temperature 63°	activity	

	2	The leading therapist introduces and explains the activity with support of the co-therapists
Comfortable seating		
Prepared structure activity	3	All members of the group participate in the activity.

OCCUPATIONAL THERAPY SERVICE

TOPIC	Loan of equipment
SUB-TOPIC	Access of community loaned equipment
STANDARD	ADL equipment supplied to patient's home environment meets the need of the patient and carer

STRUCTURE	PROCESS	OUTCOME
Referral procedure in use Access to a qualified OT A referral procedure to home loans, community stores, equipment loans is in use There is a policy for supply of equipment following BAOT guidelines (including: storage, sterilizing, maintenance, Health and Safety, delivery and collection – condemning) OT informed of new development of equipment	OT assesses the need for equipment, where indicated this may take place in the patient's own environment – without patient present The OT records the referral, the assessment outcome and recommendations The OT accesses equipment from community resources and records this All equipment issued is in safe working order OT has access to new products catalogues, demonstrations etc.	There is written evidence of response to referral in five working days of the assessment outcome and recommendations There is written evidence of referral to community resources listing the equipment to be supplied There is evidence the equipment supplied meets the patient's needs The policy for equipment supply is complied with New items of equipment are ordered The patiens and carers are able to demonstrate the safe use of equipment

OCCUPATIONAL THERAPY SERVICE

TOPIC	Home visits – home visits to patients residing within the community
STANDARD	The occupational therapist assesses the patient's functional activities within his/her own environment. Response to the referral for a home visit takes place within 5 working days

STRUCTURE	PROCESS	OUTCOME
There is a home visit policy following the BAOT guidelines	The OT assesses the patient's functional activities within the patient's own environment	Response to the referral takes place within 5 working days
There is a referral procedure in use	The OT assesses the carer's role	There is written evidence of the assessment procedure and find ings in the patient's notes
A qualified OT in post	The OT records the referral, the assessment, the outcome and recommendations in patient's notes	
		There is written evidence of the action taken and referral to other agencies is recorded

OCCUPATIONAL THERAPY SERVICE

TOPIC	Patient mobility
SUB-TOPIC	The supply of wheelchairs to patients
STANDARD	The occupational therapist assesses the patient's mobility needs. Action regarding a wheelchair is taken within 3 working days

STRUCTURE	PROCESS	OUTCOME
There is a wheelchair policy in use	1 The OT assesses the patient's needs	Wheelchair referrals are processed within 3 working days
There is a referral procedure in use	2 The OT records the referral, the assessment, the outcome and recommendations	
The following records are available	3 The OT completes the documentation for the supply of a wheelchair and cushion in accordance with the wheelchair policy	Appropriate wheelchair is supplied to increase the mobility of the patient
Patient's records (nursing and OT notes) Loans book DSA referral form	4 The OT orders the apropriate wheelchair from a designated supplier	There is written evidence of the action taken

A qualified ocupational
therapist

Equipment: 8L, 8BL,
9L wheelchair
A range of pressure-
relieving cushions is
readily available

Trent Core Standard for Palliative Care

CORE STANDARD:
Palliative Care

STANDARD REF:
Standard No 1 — Collaboration with other agencies

CARE GROUP:
Palliative Care Patients and Carers

STANDARD STATEMENT:
There is effective collaboration with other agencies, professional and voluntary providing continuity of care and support for patients, and their carers.

CRITERIA

Structure

There is evidence of specialised assessment and communication skills within the team.
The team has knowledge of, and links with, agencies that may be contacted to meet specific needs of the patient and carers.
The team are aware of the methods of referral, and correct channels of communication to contact and mobilise these agencies.

Process

A relevant team member, the patient and/or carer combine to assess the need for help from other agencies.
The team refers to, and communicates with the relevant agencies in accordance with individual need.
The agencies contacted, and reasons for referral are documented in the Care Plan.
The team continues to review the patient or carer needs, and refer to agencies for specialist advice and expertise.

Outcome

Specialist agencies were able to accept the referral, to report and liaise.
The patient and/or carer state that they were helped by the agencies involved.
Multidisciplinary team review confirms the specialist agencies effectiveness.

Measuring outcomes

The UK Department of Health paper *On the State of the Public Health* defines an outcome as any end result that is attributable to the intervention of the health services. Austin and Clark (1993) in an article

'Measures of Outcome: for Whom?' state that the phrase 'measures of outcome' is currently used to indicate the process of documentation of client improvement and achievement of treatment goals. It serves several purposes:

- to show that intervention is appropriate and effective;
- to indicate areas where service development might be required or additional resources deployed;
- to enable changes that lead to an improvement in consumer satisfaction;
- to show that a contracted service has been provided;
- to indicate the effective use of health resources.

They point out that the term means different things to different people – managers, clinicians, patients, carers and consumer groups.

Jeffrey (1993), in her discussion of content of outcome measures, observes that, although many outcome measures evaluate impairment and disability, more emphasis is needed on handicap as 'this area outlines the social effects of impairment and disability on the quality of life of the patient'.

In oncology and palliative care, the occupational therapist will be looking at residual dysfunction and deterioration in the later stages of the disease. As well as the physical dysfunction, the occupational therapist also has to consider the following, as commonly identified as quality of life issues (Doyle *et al.*, 1993):

- physical concerns – symptoms, pain;
- functional ability – activity, self-care;
- emotional well-being;
- psychological functioning;
- social functioning;
- occupational functioning;
- spirituality;
- sexuality (including body image);
- treatment satisfaction;
- financial concerns;
- future plans/orientation (for example, hope, planning);
- family well-being – emotional and physical.

Fricke (1993) states: 'It is essential for therapists to measure the outcome of their interventions' and reiterates a point made by Law (1990) by pointing out 'that therapists must first decide on the purpose of the assessment: descriptive, predictive or evaluative?'

She uses Figure 12.1 to illustrate this point:

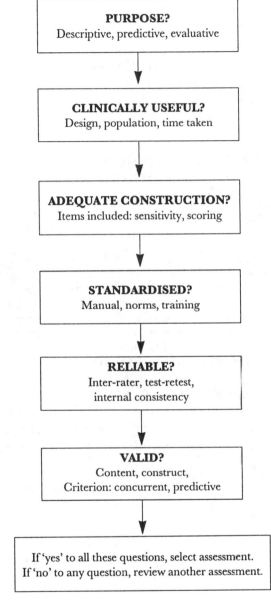

PURPOSE?
Descriptive, predictive, evaluative

CLINICALLY USEFUL?
Design, population, time taken

ADEQUATE CONSTRUCTION?
Items included: sensitivity, scoring

STANDARDISED?
Manual, norms, training

RELIABLE?
Inter-rater, test-retest,
internal consistency

VALID?
Content, construct,
Criterion: concurrent, predictive

If 'yes' to all these questions, select assessment.
If 'no' to any question, review another assessment.

Figure 12.1: The process of evaluating an assessment. Adapted from Law (1987).

The Canadian Occupational Performance Measure is an individualized measure designed to assess and evaluate the occupational performance of a client receiving occupational therapy. It reflects the goals of the client, taking into account his or her role within his or her environment. It is based on the client-centred practice of occupational therapy and uses the occupational performance model, which views the client's performance as comprising self-care, productivity and leisure. It is also founded on the belief that the client's performance is affected by an interaction of mental, physical, sociocultural and spiritual factors.

Law *et al.* (1990) describe the Canadian Occupational Performance Measure as 'an outcome measure that serves to structure and focus the asessment and intervention process . . . and [which] should be of assistance to therapists in integrating these guidelines into their clinical practice.'

As with all assessments, it does not claim to be of use in all clinical areas so therapists need to be selective. Occupational therapists require standardized and validated outcome measures to justify and prove the efficacy of their treatment interventions. However, McKenna (1992) remarks that:

> The limitations of a scientific approach to quality of life seem clear. Because people are viewed homogeneously, human behaviour is fractured into a number of quantifiable parameters and assessment tools are designed to yield only data which are precise and repeatable, the very individual and personal nature of life quality cannot be tapped. Whilst objective assessments arguably have a necessary place in our practice, Occupational Therapists must not lose sight of the value or art of seeing the individual in his or her own unique context.

Higginson (1995) discusses a range of 12 outcome measures that have been used or proposed for use in palliative care. She reinforces the point that outcome measures need to reflect the objectives of the service or treatment if they are to measure its effectiveness:

> Therefore, palliative care cannot be measured with commonly used outcome measures such as mortality or disability, but requires measurement of aspects which are important to patients with progressive disease and their families.

Examples of aspects for outcome measurement in palliative care

General areas

- Quality of life – all aspects, physical, emotional, social, spiritual.
- Quality of dying – all aspects as for quality of life but including resolving last issues, planning.
- Bereavement outcome.

Specific examples

- Control of pain and symptoms.
- Relief of anxieties and fears for patient and family.
- Meeting wishes for place of care and death (for example, at home).
- Meet needs for practical care, financial help.
- Patient and family feel that communication and information have been as they would wish.
- Last wishes before death are met – for example, meeting with estranged family.
- Satisfaction with care.
- Relief of depression.
- Lessened mortality and morbidity during bereavement.

Auditing

Higginson (1992) advises that:

> Before audit can begin the unit must decide whether to measure the quality of care in terms of its structure (the resources), process (the use of resources) or outcome (the result). Of course, a combination of these elements can be used and may be beneficial.

Examples of measures of structure, process and outcome measure in palliative care

Structure = the resources
- staffing mix, grades
- financial resources
- home care/hospital/hospice services
- day hospice places
- number of staff per cancer patient
- drugs and equipment available.

Process = the use of resources
- drugs prescribed
- number of visits
- throughput
- procedures followed
- documentation

- time taken in a visit
- equipment given out.

Outcome – the result
- symptoms
- pain
- anxiety
- needs met, e.g. requiring no more practical equipment
- resolved fears, grief, anger
- open and honest communication as the patient wishes
- wishes for place of death met
- satisfaction.

Measuring structure, process and outcome: difficulties and meaning

Structure is the easiest to measure because its elements are the most stable and identifiable. However, it is an indirect measure of the quality of care and its value depends on the nature of its influence on care (Donabedian, 1980). Structure is relevant to quality in that it increases or decreases the probability of a good performance.

Process is one step closer to changes in the health status of individuals. The advantage of process is that it measures the most immediately discernible attributes of care activities. However, it is only valuable as a measure once the elements of process are known to have a clear relationship with the desired changes in health status (Donabedian, 1980).

Outcome reflects the true change in health status, and thus is the most relevant for patients and society. However, it is difficult to eliminate other causes for change, such as prior care. A useful approach is to focus on the difference between the desired outcome and the actual outcome (Shaw, 1980). Services can then identify whether or not their goals are being achieved and investigate any failings.

Some examples of audit tools used in oncology and palliative care follow.

Royal Marsden NHS Trust Auditing Tools: Occupational Therapy Standards of Care

GENERAL STANDARD
PATIENT OPINION

The occupational therapy staff at the Royal Marsden Hospital are constantly trying to improve the service they provide for patients. It is of enormous help to have the views of patients to help us do this and we would like to collect some information from you about your experience of the care the occupational therapists have provided.

We would be very grateful if you would be willing to complete this questionnaire and return it in the envelope provided. The information you provide is confidential and will be treated accordingly.

Thank you for taking the time to complete this questionnaire

1. Were you clear about why the occupational   [ ] Yes   [ ] No
   therapist was asked to see you?

2. Did you have an opportunity to discuss your   [ ] Yes   [ ] No
   practical needs, e.g. how you would manage
   at home, with the occupational therapist?

Please comment if you would like to:

3. Did the advice, information and/or practical
   help that you received from the occupational
   therapist enable you to be more independent?

   Advice   [ ] Yes   [ ] No
                                                  [ ] Not applicable

   Information   [ ] Yes   [ ] No
                                                  [ ] Not applicable

   Practical help   [ ] Yes   [ ] No
                                                  [ ] Not applicable

   If no, what would have further helped you?

4. If you received any equipment from the
    occupational therapist,

    (a) Did you find it useful?   [ ] Yes   [ ] No
                                                  [ ] Not applicable

    (b) Did you receive enough information to
         put it to use easily?   [ ] Yes   [ ] No
                                                  [ ] Not applicable

    (c) Did you receive it promptly?   [ ] Yes   [ ] No
                                                  [ ] Not applicable

    If no, please comment as to any difficulties you had:

5. If you received any written information from
    the occupational therapist, did you find it
    understandable and helpful?

    [ ] Did not receive any written information
    Understandable   [ ] Yes   [ ] No
    Helpful   [ ] Yes   [ ] No

    If no, what would have made it more useful?

6. If you attended relaxation classes run by
    occupational therapy did you find them   [ ] Yes   [ ] No
    useful?   [ ] Not applicable

    If no, what would have made them more useful?

7. If you had a 'home visit' from the occupational
    therapist:

    (a) Did you understand the reasons for it?   [ ] Yes   [ ] No
                                                  [ ] Not applicable

    (b) Was it helpful?   [ ] Yes   [ ] No
                                                  [ ] Not applicable

    Please comment if you would like to:

8. If complications were to arise related to
   managing independently at home, do you   [ ] Yes   [ ] No
   know who to contact?

   Please comment if you would like to:

9. Overall, did you feel that the occupational
   therapist helped to prepare you for returning   [ ] Yes   [ ] No
   home?

   Please comment if you would like to:

10. Overall, were you satisfied with the advice/
    treatment offered by the occupational   [ ] Yes   [ ] No
    therapist?

    Please comment if you would like to:

11. What did you find the most helpful about the
    treatment offered by the occupational therapist?

12. What did you find the least helpful about the
    treatment offered by the occupational therapist?

    Are there any other comments you would like to make?

Thank you for taking the time to complete this questionnaire

GENERAL STANDARD
OCCUPATIONAL THERAPIST OPINION

STANDARD STATEMENT

Occupational therapy is directed towards enabling patients to achieve
and maintain their optimum level of independence in all areas of their
daily lives.

1. Did you consider that the timing of the   [ ] Yes   [ ] No
   occupational therapy was appropriate?

   If no, what information were you lacking?

2. Do you consider that you had access to all
   members of the multidisciplinary team that   [ ] Yes   [ ] No
   you required to achieve this standard?

   If not, who was not available, and how did
   this impact on the care you were aiming to
   provide?

3. Do you consider that you had access to the   [ ] Yes   [ ] No
   equipment necessary to achieve this standard?

   If no, what was not available and why?

4. Do you consider that you had access to the
   environment necessary to achieve this   [ ] Yes   [ ] No
   standard?

   If no, what was unavailable or unsuitable and why?

5. Do you consider that you had access to the
   educational and managerial support necessary
   to achieve this standard?
   Educational support   [ ] Yes   [ ] No
   Managerial support   [ ] Yes   [ ] No

   If no, what aspect(s) were not met and how did
   this impact on the care you were aiming to
   provide?

6. Do you feel that you were able to follow the   [ ] Yes   [ ] No
   professional practice described in the standard?

   If no, which sections were you unable to follow
   and why?

7. Do you consider that you received adequate
   information (via report, care plans and   [ ] Yes   [ ] No
   documentation) to maintain continuity of care
   while caring for this patient?

   If no, what information were you lacking?

8. Do you consider that the patient achieved
   their optimum level of independence?   [ ] Yes   [ ] No

   If no, why do you feel they were unable
   to achieve this?

9. Do you consider that the patient and
   family were able to manage safely and   [ ] Yes   [ ] No
   independently in the community?

   If no, please comment.

10. Do you consider that the patient was
    satisfied with their care?   [ ] Yes   [ ] No

    If no, why do you feel that the patient
    was not satisfied?

11. Overall, do you feel satisfied with the
    care that you delivered to the patient?   [ ] Yes   [ ] No

    If no, why were you not satisfied?

    Do you have any other comments you
    would like to make?

GENERAL STANDARD
DOCUMENTATION

STANDARD STATEMENT

Occupational therapy is directed towards enabling patients to achieve
and maintain their optimum level of independence in all areas of their
daily lives.

1. Is there evidence that the patient was
   contacted within 72 hours of referral?   [ ] Yes   [ ] No

2. Is there evidence that the following was
   assessed?
   (a) The patient's medical history   [ ] Yes   [ ] No

(b) The patient's view of current situation [ ] Yes [ ] No
(c) Functional ability related to ADL's [ ] Yes [ ] No
(d) Functional ability related to mobility [ ] Yes [ ] No
(e) Potential need for pressure area care [ ] Yes [ ] No
(f) Psychological state [ ] Yes [ ] No
(g) The patient's social situation [ ] Yes [ ] No

3. Were problem areas clearly listed in the
documentation? [ ] Yes [ ] No

4. Were the treatment aims reflective of the
problems identified? [ ] Yes [ ] No

5. Is there evidence that care was evaluated? [ ] Yes [ ] No

6. If outcomes were not achieved, is there [ ] Yes [ ] No
evidence of action taken? [ ] Not applicable

7. Is there evidence that at discharge the patient
had reached their maximum potential? [ ] Yes [ ] No

8. Is there evidence that at discharge the patient
and family would be able to manage [ ] Yes [ ] No
independently in the community?

9. If a formal assessment (e.g. for Social Services,
Disability Services Centre, Disablement [ ] Yes [ ] No
Resettlement Officer etc.) was necessary, was [ ] Not applicable
a written report sent to the appropriate person?

10. If referral to members of the multidisciplinary
team or community care was necessary,
(a) Was it made at an appropriate stage? [ ] Yes [ ] No
[ ] Not applicable

(b) Is there evidence that the appropriate [ ] Yes [ ] No
information was clearly communicated? [ ] Not applicable

**HOPE auditing tools, including audit of response to home visit
and wheelchair audit record.**

Audit response to home visit

Standard statement – the occupational therapist assesses the patient's
functional activities within his/her own environment. Response to the
referral for a home visit takes place within 5 working days.

The referral date and assessment date are clearly   YES/NO
documented in the patient's records

Comment:

A record of the assessment, including details
of the patient's and carer's functional   YES/NO
activities within their environment, is clearly
documented in the patient's notes

Comment:

There is written evidence of the action   YES/NO
taken, includung referral to other agencies

General comments:

Date of audit

Person conducting the audit

Number of case notes examined

Signature

Wheelchair audit record
The referral date and assessment date were   YES/NO
clearly documented in the patient's records

A period of more than 3 working days had   YES/NO
not elapsed between referral and assessment

Comment:

A clear record of the assessment is
documented on the occupational tharapy
record of wheelchair assessment form   YES/NO
which is held on the patient's records

Comment:

A clear record of the assessment and outcome
is documented in the OT notes   YES/NO

Comment:

The prescribed wheelchair is clearly labelled for
patient's use   YES/NO

Comment:

The prescribed wheelchair is available and
accessible for patient's use   YES/NO

Comment:

There is clear documentation available regarding
chair loaned to patient   YES/NO

Comment:

Every wheelchair supplied is used with an
appropriate cushion   YES/NO

Comment:

There is clear documentation regarding
pressure care and supplied appropriate   YES/NO
wheelchair cushion

Comment:

Trent Core Standard for Palliative Care

STANDARD STATEMENTS
Standard No 1 — Collaboration with other agencies

AUDIT
Outcome Audit:

1. Specialist agencies state that the referral was acceptable
and that they were enabled to report and liaise.   Yes/No

Audit from documentation
2. The patient and/or carer state that they were helped by
the agencies involved.   Yes/No
    Audit question– "did the . . . help you with your needs?"

3. Multidisciplinary team review confirms the specialist
   agencies effectiveness.   Yes/No
        Audit from documentation

Process Audit:

---

1. Is there evidence that the patient, and/or carer were
   involved in assessing the need for referral to   Yes/No
   specialist agencies?
   Audit question – "Were you involved in the decision
   to ask the . . . to see you?"

2. Were the carers' needs assessed individually?   Yes/No
   Audit question – "Were you asked if you had any
   problems?"
   "Were there any problems that you had which were
   not dealt with?"

3. Did the team refer to, and communicate with the
   relevant agencies?   Yes/No
        Audit from documentation

4. Was referral to, and involvement of the specialist
   agencies documented in the Nursing Care plan?   Yes/No

        Audit from Nursing Notes

5. Was there evidence of on-going review/anticipatory
   planning of future need for specialist agency services?   Yes/No

        Audit from Nursing Notes

Summary

In order to achieve a successful standard and auditing system the standards need to be accepted by those using them. Ownership of the standards and communication within the team are vital. In the event that change is necessary to the service it can be effectively implemented because there will be a clear understanding of what has taken place.

The advantages and disadvantages of standards need to be considered so that they are used appropriately. Different models should be considered in order to identify which is most suited to the service.

In order to audit the occupational therapy input it is necessary to establish the outcome measure that accurately reflects what the treatment has achieved. This raises complex issues as there are psychological, emotional, social, spiritual, physical and functional aspects to be considered.

Evans (1992) observes that 'introducing rigorous self-appraisal into units caring for people is not easy . . . However, in a movement committed to the philosophy of putting the patient first, introducing quality measures ensures that patients and their families will continue to get the best possible service.'

Action points

1. Outline the key points in a multidisciplinary audit on an acute oncology unit.
2. Choose a method of auditing outcomes of the occupational therapy service and establish areas in which changes can be made to that service.
3. How does standard-setting and auditing benefit the clients, the occupational therapy service and the employing authority?

References

Austin C, Clark CR (1993) Measures of outcome: for whom? British Journal of Occupational Therapy 56(1): 21–4.

Department of Health (1992) On the State of the Public Health: the Annual Report of the Chief Medical Officer 1991. London: HMSO.

Donabedian A (1966) Evaluating the quality of medical care, Part II. Milbank Memorial Fund Quarterly 44(3): 166–203.

Doyle D, Hanks GWC, MacDonald N (1993) Oxford Textbook of Palliative Medicine. Oxford: Oxford University Press.

Evans R (1992) Foreword. In National Council for Hospice and Specialist Palliative Care Services (Ed). Quality, Standards, Organisational and Clinical Audit for Hospice and Palliative Care Services. London: NCH & SPCS.

Fricke J (1993) Measuring outcomes in rehabilitation: a review. British Journal of Occupational Therapy 56(6): 217–21.

Higginson I (1992) Quality, Standards, Organisational and Clinical Audit for Hospice and Palliative Care Services. London: NCH & SPCS.

Higginson I (1995) Outcome Measures in Palliative Care. London: NCH & SPCS.

Jeffrey LIH (1993) Aspects of selecting outcome measures to demonstrate the effectiveness of comprehensive rehabilitation. BJOT 56(11): 394–400.

Kitson A (1989) Standards of Care: A Framework for Quality. London: RCN Scutari Press.

Law M (1987) Measurement in occupational therapy: scientific criteria for evaluation. Canadian Journal of Occupational Therapy 54(3): 133–8.

Law M, Baptiste S, McColl MA, Opzoomer A, Polatajko H, Pollock N (1990) The Canadian Occupational Performance Measure: an outcome measure for occupational therapy. Canadian Journal of Occupational Therapy 57(2): 82–7.

Luthert J, Robinson L (1993) The Royal Marsden Hospital Manual of Standards of Care. London: NHS Trust.

McKenna K (1993) Quality of life: A question of functional outcomes or the fulfilment of life plans. The Australian Occupational Therapy Journal 40(1) 33–5.

Nightingale Macmillan Continuing Care Unit (1992) Palliative Care Core Standards – A Multidisciplinary Approach. Derby: Derbyshire Royal Infirmary.

Sale D (1990) Quality Assurance Essentials of Nursing Management. Basingstoke: Macmillan Education Ltd.

HOPE (1993) Standards and Audit Tools. London: HOPE.

The Royal Marsden NHS Trust (1992) Standards of Care. London.

Wilson C (1987) Hospital Wide Quality Assurance: Models for Implementation and Development. Ontario: WB Saunders.

Appendix 1
Hospital Policies and Procedures

A: Priorities of Care Statement, St George's Hospital, London

The following is used by the Occupational Therapy Department at the above hospital in order to give clear guidelines to the staff on how to prioritize their busy workloads. It can also be presented to other disciplines to explain how patients are being prioritized if this is brought into question.

The Occupational Therapy department at this hospital has prepared the following statement on dealing with referrals to our service.

The following criteria provide guidelines for prioritizing referrals and work within our department during periods of staff shortage or increased rates of referrals.

High priority criteria

1. Patients living alone without support who are at risk in the home environment.
2. Patients with a carer who is unable to provide the necessary support and has no support from community services.
3. Patients with a limited life expectancy who are to return home.
4. Patients who without occupational therapy intervention would incur deformity and/or loss of function.
5. Patients who would be unable to carry out ADL without occupational therapy intervention and where assistance is not available.

NB In patients have priority over out patients.

Low priority criteria

1. Patients living with supportive relatives/carers and who have support from community services.
2. Patients who fail to attend appointments and who are not at risk (at discretion of Occupational Therapist).
3. Patients who refuse treatment and who are not at risk (at discretion of Occupational Therapist).
4. Patients who are awaiting alternative accommodation and who are in hospital.
5. Patients who could attend occupational therapy after discharge and who can manage at home.

Administrative duties

1. Patient assessment and treatment.
2. Reports, note-writing, statistics (must be documented within 24 hours).
3. Liaison with other professionals.
4. Health and safety check.
5. Staff supervision.
6. Stock control.
7. Finance – ordering/petty cash.

Reproduced by kind permission of Occupational Therapy Department, St George's Hospital, London.

B: Typical Procedures for Loan of Equipment: Occupational Therapy Department

1. **Introduction**
1.1 Department equipment to aid independent living is primarily for assessment use within the hospital setting.
1.2 Equipment from the occupational therapy department is for loan by occupational therapy staff only.
1.3 Following assessment of the patient by an occupational therapist, the appropriate item of equipment may be loaned for the patient to use whilst in hospital.

2. **Wheelchairs**
2.1 Refer to Hospital Policy relating to assessment for and loan of wheelchairs.
2.2 The occupational therapist assesses for and may loan a department wheelchair, and sends the patient's local wheelchair

service a written request for replacement of the wheelchair and pressure cushion.

2.3 In the event that a patient needs to take an occupational therapy department wheelchair home, the carers must undertake to return the wheelchair to the hospital when it is no longer in use.

2.4 Wheelchairs from the occupational therapy department are not for purchase by any patients. A list of suppliers is available for both sites, both to rent and buy.

2.5 Wheelchairs are not available to loan out to patients to keep in their own home for shopping outings or just occasional use.

3.   Pressure cushions

3.1 Each occupational therapy department has a supply of pressure cushions for assessment and use in the hospital.

3.2 The pressure cushion must be thoroughly cleaned after use by a patient before being reissued to another patient.

3.3 The cushions are for use in hospital and not to be loaned out to the community. This is the responsibility of the community services, e.g. district nursing or Macmillan nursing services. If they do not have access to appropriate pressure cushions, each individual case can be assessed as necessary.

3.4 Assessments and prescriptions for pressure cushions should be sent off to wheelchair centres together with wheelchair forms as appropriate.

4.   Bathing and toileting equipment

4.1 Equipment to assist patients with toileting or bathing may be loaned following assessment by the occupational therapist.

4.2 It is the professional decision of the occupational therapist whether it is appropriate to loan it from the department or whether the patient can wait for social services to provide it. This is influenced by the distance the patient lives from the hospital and whether carers will be able to return it.

4.3 Patients and carers must be shown how to fit and use equipment safely and correctly. Written information is available in the department to complement this.

5.   Kitchen and minor items of equipment

5.1 . . . equipment to assist patients for their use in hospital or short term outpatient use may be loaned following assessment by the occupational therapist.

5.2 The occupational therapist should prepare a functional report identifying equipment required and send this to the patient's local social services occupational therapy service. They will inform this hospital of the availability of equipment and which items they provide.

5.3 If the social services department does not provide small items, the patient and/or carer will need to purchase them.

5.4 The occupational therapist can provide an appropriate catalogue regarding provision of equipment.

5.5 Small, portable items of equipment, e.g. kettles, iron, even ovens are not to be loaned out at all . . .

6. **On loans forms**

6.1 If large pieces of equipment are to be loaned for use outside the hospital, fill in an on loans form or the appropriate folder in the occupational therapy department.

6.2 Give the patient/carer our contact number should they need help in returning or having it collected.

* * * * * *

Appendix 2
Stairlifts

Prepared by the Occupational Therapy Department, The Royal Marsden NHS Trust, London. The following illustrates a patient information sheet that explains the principles to consider when privately purchasing a stairlift and how to contact representatives of different companies. It also emphasizes that no bias is being given to any particular company.

'Stairlifts are powered lifts mounted on stair-fixed tracks which follow the line of the stairs. The track can usually be sited on either side of the stairs and both curved and straight tracks are available. Three types of stairlift can be used in the domestic setting:

– seated stairlift, standing stairlift and stairlifts with a wheelchair platform.'

Disabled Living Foundation

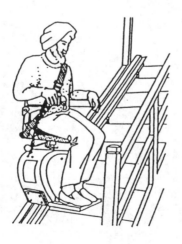

Seated stairlift

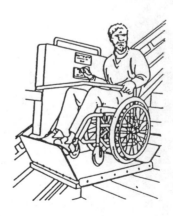

Wheelchair platform

There are various companies dealing in stairlifts, all have regional advisers who will visit you at home to assess your stairs and advise on suitable products. A few are listed below but not necessarily recommended by this hospital.

Addresses of appropriate companies

The following company sells new and reconditioned stairlifts and also purchases second-hand ones.

Addresses of appropriate companies

* * * * * *

Appendix 3 Occupational Therapy Measurement Form for Furniture

Prepared by the Occupational Therapy Department, St George's Hospital, London. The following shows a form on which patients' relatives can measure and record furniture heights for ordering equipment. This is used when clear explanations concerning the correct use of equipment have already been given to the realtives during the occupational therapy assessment.

**OCCUPATIONAL THERAPY
MEASUREMENT FORM FOR FURNITURE**

Patient's Name:
Occupational Therapist:

Please measure the following:

CHAIR
Usual chair: Height when sat on _____
*castors/wooden legs
Other chair: Height when sat on _____
*castors/wooden legs

BED
Height when sat on _____   *double/single
Number of legs _____   *legs with castors
*wooden legs
*others specify

TOILET
Height of pan only _____
Position of rails (if any) _____

BATH
Overall width across top _____ *enamel/acrylic
Position of rails (if any) _____

Appendix 4
Form for Assessing Upper-Limb Dysfunction

Adapted by the Occupational Therapy Department, The Royal Marsden NHS Trust. The following form shows the key areas to be assessed and recorded by the occupational therapist in the assessment of upper-limb dysfunction.

ASSESSMENT OF CLIENTS WITH UPPER-LIMB DYSFUNCTION

Name   Hospital no
Age   Consultant

Diagnosis

History

Dominant hand   limb(s) affected

Main problems (as identified by client)

Main difficulties at home

Attitude to disability

Range of movement	
Shoulder	
Elbow	
Wrist	
Hand	
Sensory	

MANIPULATION		COMMENTS
Light pinch	Pick up pencil – write name	
Heavy pinch	Strike match Do up zip	
Tripod grip	lift lid of saucepan Small screwdriver	
Grasp	Hold mug Lift full kettle	
Opposition	Do up buttons Wind watch	
Pronation/ Supination	Screw jam jar Turn key in lock	
Miscellaneous	Handle money Pick up telephone Carry bag	

	ACTIVITIES OF DAILY LIVING
PADL Washing Dressing Grooming	
DADL Food preparation/ cooking Washing Shopping Cleaning	

SUMMARY

NEEDS

ACTION TAKEN

Signature   Date

DATE FOR REVIEW

Appendix 5
Wheelchair Cushion Referral Forms

Prepared by the Wheelchair Service, Merton and Sutton NHS Wheelchair Trust, Surrey. The form is used by the occupational therapist in the assessment and prescription of pressure-relief cushions.

PRESSURE RELIEVING WHEELCHAIR CUSHION REFERRAL FORM

Return form to:

Name of client..

D.O.B..................... Sex M/F

Address...

Height..................... Weight..........

....

.............................Postcode....................

Indicate if any recent weight changes

Telephone no:..

Gain...................... Loss..............

GP (Name and telephone no)

....

Carer/Parent (Name and telephone no)

....

Does client live on own: YES/NO

Diagnosis and recent history of pressure problems: (inc. diabetic, incontinence etc.)

....

....

General Health   Stable..........   Poor..........   Deteriorating..........

Where is site of pressure problem?

Left ischial...............   right ischial.................   left trochanter................

right trochanter................   sacrum................   other (specify)................

What grade is the sore? –

superficial................... deep................... involving bone...................

Is the sore being treated?   Yes/No   If 'yes' by whom

Is nurse visiting? daily.......... weekly.......... occasionally.......... no..........

Is client able to adjust position to relieve pressure? ....

Is client able to maintain a symmetrical position? ....

Average number of hours per day of continuous sitting in wheelchair ....

WATERLOW PRESSURE SORE PREVENTION / TREATMENT POLICY

RING SCORES IN TABLE, ADD TOTAL. SEVERAL SCORES PER CATEGORY CAN BE USED.

BUILD/WEIGHT FOR HEIGHT	*	SKIN TYPE VISUAL RISK AREAS	*	SEX AGE	*	SPECIAL RISKS	*
						TISSUE MALNUTRITION	*
AVERAGE	0	HEALTHY	0	MALE	1	E.G.: TERMINAL CACHEXIA	8
ABOVE AVERAGE	1	TISSUE PAPER	1	FEMALE	2	CARDIAC FAILURE	5
OBESE	2	DRY	1	14–49	1	PERIPHERAL VASCULAR	5
BELOW AVERAGE	3	OEDEMATOUS	1	50–64	2	DISEASE	
		CLAMMY (TEMP)	1	65–74	3	ANAEMIA	2
CONTINENCE	*	DISCOLOURED	1	75–80	4	SMOKING	1
		BROKEN/SPOT	1	81+	5		
COMPLETE/ CATHETERISED	0					NEUROLOGICAL DEFICIT	*
OCCASION INCONT	1	MOBILITY	*	APPETITE	*	E.G.: DIABETES, M.S, CVA,	4–6
CATH/INCONT OF FAECES	2	FULLY	0	AVERAGE	0	MOTOR/SENSORY PARAPLEGIA	
DOUBLY INCONT	3	RESTLESS/		POOR	1		
		FIDGETY	1	N.G. TUBE/		MAJOR SURGERY/TRAUMA	*
		APATHETIC	2	FLUIDS ONLY	2		
		RESTRICTED	3	NBM/		ORTHOPAEDIC -	
		INERT/TRACTION	4	ANOREXIC	3	BELOW WAIST SPINAL	5
						ON TABLE> 2 HOURS	5

SCORE	10+ AT RISK	15+ HIGH RISK	20+ VERY HIGH RISK

MEDICATION	*
CYTOTOXICS, HIGH DOSE STEROIDS ANTI - INFLAMMATORY	4
Total	

© J Waterlow 1991 Revised March 1992
OBTAINABLE FROM: NEWTONS, CURLAND, TAUNTON, TA3 5SG

Date Waterlow score was taken ..../.............../...............

What pressure relieving product is clint now on:-

(i)   Bed..   (ii)   Wheelchair..................................

(iii)   Armchair......................................   (iv)   Other..

Other products tried: Reason for rejection:

....

....

....

....

Referred by (print name):......................   Date:..

Address:..   Tel. No:..

....

...................................Post Code:............

Therapist recommendation.   W.S. only

Cushion model...................   size....................   cover...................

Reason for selection..

Therapist's signature..   Date..

GUIDELINES FOR THE TRAINED PROFESSIONALS WHEN SELECTING (PRESSURE PREVENTION) CUSHIONS FOR WHEELCHAIR USERS IN MERTON & SUTTON COMMUNITY NHS TRUST

Desc. & properties	Additional comments	AT RISK	HIGH RISK	VERY HIGH RISK
COVERS FOR ALL CUSHIONS Fabric has significant effect on pressure	i Two-way stretch terry towelling ii Dartex or similar Both reduced pressure compared to non-stretch vinyl cover. Platilon appropriate for waterproof protection	10+ - Ability to change position - No previous history of pressure sores - Stable condition - General health good	Waterlow Scale for Guideline 15+ - Limited ability to change position - Variable condition - Long periods of sitting - Signs of redness	20+ - Immobile - Long periods sitting - Possible weight loss - General health variable to poor
FOAM Standard Temper foam Cold moulded Latex Combination	* Provides comfort * Lightweight * Easy to care * Low cost * Depth affects comfort & pressure relief * Regular turning delays deterioration * most effective on flat surfaces eg infill/crescent * replacement required when signs of bottoming- out * dependent on use and weight of user	Standard 3" Latex Dunlopillo Sunmate Polyfoam	Minimum 3" Foam & castellation Nestor Pudgee Q Care Ultimate	Ultimate Super Contour

Desc. & properties	Additional comments	AT RISK	HIGH RISK	VERY HIGH RISK
GEL Fluid gel Gel pad Gel and foam	Weight of cushion significant and may reduce propelling ability * Initial chill on sitting * some models heat to over body temperature * Care required for fluid gel * Shaped gel provides stability if postural problems	Dynamic for Posture	Primenest Bioform Sumed 93 Sumed 90 Dynamic	Jay Medical Ergonest Dynamic plus
AIR i Flotation ii Alternating	Good pressure relief if properly adjusted * over-inflation increases shear * Alternating has additional battery pack * Contraindicated if user/carer unable to adjust	Minimax Roho Low Profile Roho Nexus Roho	Low Profile Roho Enhancer if postural instability	I Roho range II Talley B.A.S.E. + Power Pack
BEDS/MATTRESS AVOID 1 Plastic draw sheets 2 Inco-pads 3. Tightly tucked-in sheets or duvet cover	Overlays or Specialist Mattressing	Alternating pressure overlays or mattresses/bed systems	Low Airloss, Bead or Alternating bed systems	

Appendix 6
Driving Guidelines

Driving guidelines. Prepared by the Occupational Therapy Department, The Royal Marsden NGS Wheelchair Trust, Surrey. The following patient information sheet highlights key areas that the patient should consider concerning returning to driving.

Occupational Therapy Department Driving

Speak to medical staff regarding how your disability will affect your ability to drive.

You are required to notify the DVLA as soon as you are aware you have a disability which is likely to last more than three months and which is or may become likely to affect your ability to drive. Your licence may not be withdrawn, but the DVLA will review your situation. For further advice, contact:

You are also obliged to contact your insurance company to notify them of your current situation and disability.

Issue of ORANGE BADGES is via local authorities. You may be eligible if you:

- receive Disabled Living Allowance (Mobility Supplement)
- are blind or
- have a permanent and substantial disability making walking difficult or impossible
- have very severe upper limb dysfunction and drive.

Badges are issued for three years, there may be a small charge. Contact your local authority for further advice and an application form.

Driving Assessment and Mobility Centres offer advice on car adaptations and all aspects of public and private transport for disabled users, there is usually a charge for assessment. See your local phone book for address and tel. no. Some useful addresses:

* * * * * *

Appendix 7
Energy Conservation

Energy conservation. Adapted by the Occupational Therapy Department, The Royal Marsden Hospital, London. The following patient advice sheet emphasizes the main areas to which patients should give consideration in reorganizing and planning their lifestyle. The aim is for them to use their energy more efficiently and avoid becoming overtired.

Energy conservation is:

- Doing a task in the shortest possible time.
- Using the least amount of energy in the most efficient way to do a good job with time left over to spend pleasurably.

There is no one way of doing a task that will be acceptable to all people.

The following advice provides suggestions for various methods of organizing and doing tasks.

Before commencing a task decide whether:

- it should be done;
- it can be given to someone else;
- it can be made easier.

Four ways of achieving energy conservation are:

1. Elimination, establishing whether all or part of the activity can be eliminated – for example, by cooking a meal in the same dish in which it will be served.

2. Changing order – energy can be conserved by carrying out activities in a different order.
3. Combining, for example collecting all articles together for a task before starting it.
4. Simplification, for example using convenience items or foods to save energy.

Principles to be aware of whilst performing a task include:

1. Avoid unnecessary exertion or rushing.
2. Avoid twisting movements – make sure your work is placed directly in front of you.
3. Avoid maintaining one posture for a prolonged length of time – e.g. standing to work, making sure you are in a comfortable position with the work surface at the correct height.
4. Avoid excessive bending – bend from the knees and not straight from the waist.
5. Avoid pushing or pressing against resistance. If you have to push then use the whole body rather than muscular effort.
6. When heavy articles have to be moved use a trolley or the assistance of another person.
7. Avoid working with arms extended or unsupported. Keep the work close to your body.

Planning and organization

Write yourself a list of activities or tasks which you wish to do, and then divide them into:

1. Daily tasks, e.g. meal preparation, making beds, washing dishes.
2. Weekly tasks, e.g. cleaning, ironing, shopping.
3. Monthly and odd interval tasks, e.g. cleaning windows.

By making a plan of what you do, you can organize your day so that you are not overloaded with work.

* * * * * *

Appendix 8
Relaxation

Appendices 8–12 are all concerned with relaxation. They were adapted by the Occupational Therapy Department, The Royal Marsden NHS Trust, London, for relaxation exercises specific to their patients. The following guidelines for assessment and treatment in the relaxation sessions enable the occupational therapist to give clear explanations to the patient, carry out assessment and treatment, and to record the outcomes.

Relaxation aims to help you:

1. To understand and recognize your level of anxiety.
2. To understand the need for relaxation and recognize certain situations that may trigger tension.
3. To experience a variety of relaxation techniques thus enabling you to choose the most appropriate.
4. To appreciate the importance of planning time for relaxation as part of your daily activities and lifestyle.
5. To improve quality of sleep.
6. To lessen pain caused by inappropriate muscle tension.
7. To encourage peace of mind.
8. To improve performance of physical skills.
9. To increase self-esteem and confidence.
10. To ease relationships with others.
11. To channel and control effects of anxiety.
12. To avoid unnecessary fatigue.

Relaxation sessions can be arranged to coincide with your other hospital appointments. These usually take place in the occupational therapy department.

* * * * * *

Appendix 9
Relaxation:
Assessment and
Treatment Plan

Name:........................ No:............... Date:.....................

Do you know why you have been referred to Occupational Therapy for relaxation?

How does anxiety affect you?

Do you suffer any of the following symptoms?

Physical	*Psychological*
tense muscles	apprehension
tension headaches	loss of confidence
dizziness	short temper
stomach churning	self consciousness
restlessness	fears
shaking	insomnia
excessive fatigue	depression
palpitations	irritability
blackouts	sexual difficulties
tightness in throat	phobias
and chest	difficulty in personal
excessive sweating	relationships
stammering	difficulty formulating thought

(cont.)

Appendix 9 continued

Current treatment – medical and other agencies involved:

How have you been coping until now?

Previous experience of relaxation:

Family history of illness:

Employment:

Expectations of relaxation:

Plan:

* * * * * *

Appendix 10
Format of Relaxation and Stress-Management Sessions

Week 1

Introduction

- explain aims of stress management
- dates of sessions
- use of tapes
- reinforce need for regular attendance and practice

Discussion re. 'what is anxiety?' and 'why use relaxation?'

Practical

Quick relaxation technique – balloon exercise

Breathing exercise

Homework: practise breathing exercise as on handout

Practise balloon exercise

Recognize physical symptoms of anxiety in different situations

Week 2

Feedback from Week 1 and its homework

Discussion

The spiral effect of anxiety

Trigger points for muscular tension

Practical

Complete body chart before and after relaxation session

Progressive muscular relaxation

Homework

Practise progressive muscular relaxation

Complete body charts in conjunction with relaxation

Week 3

Feedback from week 2 and its homework

Discussion re. ways to relax in daily activities – brainstorm

Practical

Relaxation using imagery

Choose two activities to use to relax and record

Homework

Practise relaxation using imagery

Use of handout by completing chosen activities

Week 4

Feedback from week 3 and homework

Discussion

Use of cancer support groups

Addresses for tapes and further information

Purpose of evaluation of relaxation training programme

Practical

Auto-suggestion technique

Issue evaluation forms and reply envelopes

Homework

Continued use of material in daily routine

* * * * * *

Appendix 11
Relaxation
Evaluation Form

Occupational Therapy Department
Relaxation Training

Name .... Date ....

Shade in areas on **both** sketches where you feel tense.

1. **Before relaxation session**

   Comments:

Technique used:

2. **After relaxation session**

   Comments:

Name .... Date ....

Using the scale below, circle the appropriate number for questions 1 to 3

1. **How relaxed am I as a person?**

0........ 1........ 2........ 3........ 4........ 5........ 6........ 7........ 8........ 9........ 10

Completely   Only   Never
relaxed – no   slightly   relaxed –
physical symptoms   anxious   many
                                                                     physical
                                                                     symptoms

2. **How tense do you feel before relaxation session?**

0........ 1........ 2........ 3........ 4........ 5........ 6........ 7........ 8........ 9........ 10

Not tense   Slightly   Completely
                                    tense   tense

3. **How relaxed do you feel after the session?**

Technique used: ....

0........ 1........ 2........ 3........ 4........ 5........ 6........ 7........ 8........ 9........ 10

Completely   Slightly   Completely
relaxed   relaxed   tense

Comments:

Relaxation evaluation

1. Do you feel that your original expectations were met?
2. Is there anything that you feel was not covered during the sessions?
3. What aspects did you find most helpful?
4. What aspects did you find least helpful?
5. What relaxation technique did you find the most useful (if any)?
6. Any suggested changes or recommendations for future relaxation training groups?
7. Do you feel you need any more information?

Date ....

* * * * * *

Appendix 12 Breathing Exercises and Relaxation Techniques

Breathing exercises

The following controlled breathing exercises may help you reduce symptoms of anxiety.

The exercises can be used on their own or with another relaxation technique.

Throughout these exercises, breathing should be without strain or discomfort.

Before you begin, loosen any tight clothing, position yourself comfortably, lying or sitting, and close your eyes.

* Place your hand flat on your stomach.
* Inhale deeply through your nose and take in enough air to expand your chest and stomach.
* Feel your hand move as your stomach rises.
* Exhale slowly through your mouth, emptying your lungs to flatten your chest and stomach.
* Feel your hand move as your stomach lowers.
* Pause.
* Repeat several times.

Try to establish a regular breathing pattern. It may help to try the following:

As you inhale, count slowly to a count of 4:
inhale, 2, 3, 4;
exhale, 2, 3, 4.

As you inhale, try saying a positive word or phrase, such as: 'I am relaxed', 'I am peaceful', 'I have confidence', and so forth.

Relaxation technique

This can be carried out either on its own or as part of a relaxation session with another technique, for example after 'breathing'.

This technique can be carried out while standing or seated. When standing, you may use the back of a chair for support. You may want to take off your shoes for comfort.

Your eyes may be open or closed (whichever you find most comfortable).

- Begin by concentrating on your posture.
- Relax your shoulders and knees but make sure you do not slouch.
- •• Imagine a large helium or gas-filled balloon is attached by a string to the top of your head.
- •• As the balloon rises allow it to take all the tension from your body.
- •• Acknowledge any thoughts and allow them to pass.
- Focus your mind again on the balloon and you spine as it lengthens. (Pause then, repeat from ••).
- When you are ready, let go of the balloon, return to the room and open your eyes.

Occupational therapists can use appropriate scripts for any relaxation technique – for example, progressive muscular relaxation, imagery, auto-suggestion. Clients should be reminded not to do certain exercises, such as curling toes, if they cause cramp or discomfort. If there are any external distractions or noises, advise the client to be aware of the noises around them, let them enter their mind, acknowledge them and let them drift away.

Progressive muscular relaxation

Script

(// = pause and * = repeat once)

Find a comfortable position either sitting or lying. Loosen any tight clothing and remove your shoes if you wish. Close your eyes.

Just breathe in and out deeply and slowly – in and out – in and out.//

Try to maintain this rhythm of breathing throughout.//

Try to relax to the best of your ability.//

This exercise will involve tensing and relaxing individual muscle groups.

To begin:

* Concentrate on your feet.// Curl your toes hard and point your feet away from your body.// Feel the tension in your feet//Hold the tension as you breathe in// and as you breathe out. Relax the muscles.// Just let the tension go.//

* Now press your heels hard into the bed or floor and point your feet towards your body.// Feel the tension in your ankles.// Hold the tension as you breathe in// and as you breathe out. Relax.//

* Tense your calf muscles.// Feel the tension in your calves.// Hold the tension as you breathe in// and as you breathe out.// Relax the muscles.// Just let the tension go.//

* Straighten your knees and tense the thigh muscles.// Feel the tension in your legs.// Hold the tension as you breathe in// and as you breathe out. Relax.//

* Pull in your stomach muscles.// Make your stomach feel hard, pull in the muscles firmly.//Feel the tension in your stomach and// hold the tension as you breathe in// and as you breathe out// relax the muscles// just let the tension go.//

* Make a fist with both hands.// Feel the tension in your fingers and wrists and// hold the tension as you breathe in// and as you breathe out// relax the muscles// straighten your fingers and let the tension go.//

* Press the palms of the hands hard into the bed or the chair.// Feel the tension as it moves up your arms.// Hold the tension as you breathe in// and as you breathe out.// Relax the muscles.//

* Hunch up your shoulders and press your head hard back into the pillow or chair.// Feel the tension in your neck, shoulders and head.// Hold the tension as you breathe in// and as you breathe out.// Relax the muscles.// Pull down your shoulders and let the tension go.//

* Tense the muscles of your face and jaw.// Make a frown, screw up your eyes.//Feel the tension in your face, across your forehead.// Hold the tension as you breathe in// and as you breathe out.// Relax the muscles.// Make your face feel smooth.// Straighten the lines and let the tension go.//

Be aware of the feeling of relaxation in your arms and legs.//

You are lying heavy and relaxed, warm and comfortable.//

Enjoy this feeling of relaxation for a while and listen to the music that supports the relaxation.//

[Music.]

It is now time to draw this relaxation to a close.//

Begin to become aware of the noises around you. Slowly bring yourself back to the room.//

When you are ready, slowly stretch your arms, legs and back, open your eyes and slowly sit up.

Relaxation using Imagery: 'the Beach'

Script

(//=pause)

Find a comfortable position, either sitting or lying. Loosen any tight clothing and remove your shoes if you wish. Close your eyes.

[Begin with a breathing exercise.]//

Just try to relax to the best of your ability.//

As you lie there feeling relaxed and easy, imagine yourself walking along a beach. It is a beautiful, warm, sunny day and the sky above you is dotted with white fluffy clouds.//

Try to imagine the sound of waves coming in and out,// in and out,// and the sound of the sea birds overhead.//

As the beach stretches out in front of you, you notice the warm, soft, golden colour of the sand.//

In the distance, you notice a large rock.// Its outline is blurred by a mist drifting in from over the sea.// The air smells fresh – of the ocean.//

And as you continue to wander along the beach// you feel the gentle breeze on your face and hair.// The air is cool and gentle as it strokes your face and hair.//

As you walk towards the sea// you notice the cool fresh feeling of the water as it rushes across your feet.//

As you walk along feeling perfectly relaxed and carefree, enjoy this feeling of freedom and calmness.//

You wander further along the beach and you notice a large sand dune in the distance. Walk towards it and climb to the top.//

The sand feels soft and inviting beneath your feet.// You are safe and secure.// Find a place nestled quietly amongst the dunes and lie down.//

The sand is warm under your body// you feel yourself sinking into it// feeling heavy and relaxed.// As you sink into the sand, feel its warmth on the back of your head,// shoulders,// arms// and legs.//

In the distance, hear the sound of the waves coming in and out,// in and out,// and feel the warmth of the sun on your body// as you lie there perfectly relaxed and supported in the sand.//

You do not have a care in the world.//

This is a special place for you.//

You can visit this place in your mind whenever you choose to.//

This is a place where you feel calm,// relaxed,// and secure,// free from tension and worries.//

Enjoy this feeling for a while and listen to the music which supports the relaxation.//

It is now time to return from your special place.//

Begin to become aware of the noises around you. Slowly bring yourself back to the room.

In a moment, you will get up feeling refreshed and relaxed.

When you are ready, slowly stretch your arms, legs and back, open your eyes and sit up.

Relaxation using auto-suggestion

Script

(//=pause)

Find a comfortable position either sitting or lying. Loosen any tight clothing and remove your shoes if you wish.

Take three deep breaths// and then breathe freely// and try to control the rhythm of your breathing. I will talk to you in the first person, and while listening to me, imagine my voice as you, speaking to yourself. Please do not think of anything else; listen only to the words which I say to you. Experience complete internal rest.

We shall begin . . .

I am lying very comfortably.//

Very comfortably.//

I close my eyes.//

I relax all my muscles.//

I breathe easily and regularly and without difficulty.//

Everything is of minor importance.//

Nothing is bothering me.//

I am not thinking of anything.//

I experience peace.//

I relax the muscles of my right arm.//

My right arm is becoming heavy.//

Very heavy.

I cannot lift it.//

I relax the muscles of my left arm.//

My left arm becomes heavy.//

Very heavy.

I cannot lift it.//

I breathe lightly, regularly and without difficulty.//

I relax the muscles of my right leg.//

My leg is becoming heavy.//

Very heavy.

I cannot lift it.//

I relax the muscles of my left leg.//

My leg is becoming so heavy.//

Very heavy.

It is so heavy that I cannot lift it.//

I breathe deeply, regularly and without difficulty.//

I relax the muscles of my neck, face and head.//

My head rests peacefully without tension.//

It becomes heavy.//

My whole body is relaxed in a pleasant way and I am unable to move.//

I experience peace.//

Warmth goes through my right arm.//

I feel it more and more distinctly.//

My arm is getting warmer and warmer.//

Warmth goes through my left arm.//

I experience it more and more distinctly.//

My arm is getting warmer and warmer.//

Warmth goes through my right leg.//

I feel it more and more distinctly.//

My leg is getting warmer and warmer.//

Warmth goes through my left leg.//

I experience it more and more distinctly.//

My leg is getting warmer and warmer.//

From my arms, the warmth passes into the chest.//

And from my legs, the warmth moves into my abdomen.//

Warmth is now circulating throughout my whole body.//

My whole body is warm as though I am having a warm bath.//

I feel relaxed.//

I feel great internal rest.//

I feel safe, relaxed and peaceful.//

I am taking care of myself.//

I am worthy of care.//

I approve of myself.//

I am safe.//

This peace and these thoughts will remain with me.//

They will give me power and self-assurance.//

I feel now like a person who awakes after a healthy restoring peace.//

The feeling of inability to move disappears.//

I stretch my hands, legs and back.//

I open my eyes.//

I feel light.//

I feel well.

* * * * * *

Appendix 13
Useful Addresses

Occupational therapy

Britain

UK College of Occupational
Therapists
6–8 Marshalsea Road
London
SE1 1HL
UK

United States

American Occupational
Therapy Association Inc.
4720 Montgomery Lane
PO Box 31220
Bethesda
MD 20824-1220
USA

Canada

The Canadian Association of
Occupational Therapists
Carleton Technology and
Training Centre
Suite 3400
Carleton University Campus
1125 Colonel By Drive
Ottawa
K15 5R1
Canada

Oncology and palliative care

United Kingdom

BACUP
3 Bath Place
Rivington Street
London
EC2A 3JR
UK

Brain Tumour Foundation
PO Box 162
New Malden
Surrey
KT3 3YN,
UK

Cancerlink
17 Britannia Street
London
WC1N 9JN
UK

Cancer Relief Macmillan
Fund
15/19 Britten Street
London
SW3 3TZ
UK

Marie Curie Cancer Care
28 Belgrave Square
London
SW1X 8QG
UK

United States

National Brain Tumor
Foundation
323 Geary Street
Suite 510
San Francisco
CA 94102
USA

American Cancer Society Inc.
1599 Clifton Road NE
Atlanta
GA 30329
USA

National Cancer Institute
National Institutes of Health
Bethesda
Maryland
MD 20892
USA

National Coalition for Cancer
Survivalship
323 8th Street SW
Albuquerque
NM 87102
USA

National Hospice
Organization
1901 North Fort Myer Drive
Suite 901
Arlington
VA 22209
USA

Canada

Cancer Information Service
755 Concession Street
Hamilton
Ontario
L8V 1C4
Canada

Canadian Cancer Society
10 Alcorn Avenue
Suite 200
Toronto
Ontario
M4V 3B1
Canada

Canadian Palliative Care
Association
43 Bruyere Street
Suite 286
Ottawa
Ontario
K1N 5CB
Canada

* * * * * *

Appendix 14
Case Studies and
Discussion Points

Case study 1

Mr B is a 43-year-old gentleman with a two-and-a-half year history of multiple myeloma. He is married with no children and works as a systems analyst. He has been known to the oncology unit since diagnosis and has developed a good rapport with the medical and nursing staff. Other disciplines had not become involved as he was coping well and had needed very little time off work.

Three months ago he developed left foot drop, was seen by the physiotherapist as an outpatient for exercise and fitted with an ankle-foot orthosis. He wore this inside his shoe to help compensate for the foot drop. A CT scan showed spinal involvement which was treated by outpatient radiotherapy.

He continued to work and drive his automatic car and did not require any walking aid. His wife attended radiotherapy and physiotherapy sessions with him. They appeared positive and discussed the setback openly.

One month ago, Mr B experienced severe lower back pain and was unable to get in or out of bed or the car without his wife having to lift him. They struggled for two days in this way until his wife called in the GP. The GP immediately had him admitted to the oncology unit where spinal cord compression at T6 was diagnosed. A further course of radiotherapy was started in an effort to alleviate the pain and relieve the compression.

The occupational therapist and the physiotherapist worked jointly to assess and provide the wheelchair, seating, and transfer techniques. Mr B could tolerate sitting out of bed for up to two hours and the occupational therapist worked with the wife and client to establish a routine for washing and dressing. He was incontinent of urine and faeces, had a urinary catheter *in situ* and the nursing staff co-ordinated his care, incorporating a toileting routine for his bowels.

He and his wife did not demonstrate any strong reactions initially and Mr B, in particular, appeared pragmatic and expressed the opinion that this was another hurdle to overcome. His wife spent most of the day at the hospital with him, attended his radiotherapy and physiotherapy treatment sessions and assisted the occupational therapist in self-care practice. After eight days in hospital Mr B had good dynamic sitting balance but was paraplegic and still had no bowel or urinary control. His upper limb strength was good and he was able to transfer from bed to wheelchair using a sliding/transfer board. He could roll from side to side in bed to have a bed bath, and he transferred in and out of the bath using a bathboard and bathseat. Physically, therefore, he required minimum help in self-cares and transfers.

The ward staff suggested to his wife that she have a rest from visiting the hospital all day as she appeared tired, but she chose not to do so. She was helpful and supportive to the other patients in the ward.

Although Mr B's pain was relieved, there was no restoration of function as a result of the radiotherapy. Mr B was, therefore, referred to the palliative care team who explained their role in continuing care and symptom control as opposed to curative treatment. Mr and Mrs B had both expected this and they accepted the fact that the treatment had not been successful. They were keen to discuss Mr B's return home. A family conference was held to establish future plans.

The occupational therapist visited the wife at home without Mr B in order to assess the feasibility of his returning home to live on the ground floor. The district nurse also attended to discuss what service she would provide and how often she would need to call. It was decided that the large lounge would be used as his bedroom area and, as the WC was inaccessible, a commode would be provided. In order to separate the living area and the bedroom area, the wife asked if a screen could be provided. The occupational therapist agreed. When the district nurse began to discuss other home carers who could attend to avoid the wife needing to do all the work, Mrs B suddenly focused on the provision of the screen and commode as a matter of the utmost urgency and became very angry. She firmly refused any outside help and was adamant that she only needed the equipment and the visits from the district nurse.

When she visited the hospital after this, her attitude changed towards the staff. Mrs B was angry and used different issues to focus on depending on the member of staff. Mr B also became impatient to return home and the multidisciplinary team felt that Mr and Mrs B were unreasonable in the complaints they made regarding delay in discharge planning because transport arrangements, follow-up appointments and continuing care in the community needed to be organized.

Once the equipment was provided at home, Mr B returned home, his wife still refusing any help other than the district nurse to check and flush the catheter and oversee his general care. Although Mrs B was becoming tired, she would not accept any hospice home-care services or counselling, and contact with the oncology unit, the palliative care service and any continuing care was declined.

The occupational therapist tried to follow up to ensure the equipment was satisfactory and transfer techniques were still appropriate, but the reply was curt and no further help was wanted.

Discussion points

1. Could the team have foreseen this sudden reaction by the client and his wife?
2. Was the client and wife's acceptance of the situation in hospital taken for granted?
3. What support could be provided for the district nurse by the palliative care service, given that she was the only health care professional allowed in?
4. What future needs could the occupational therapist plan for based on her existing assessment and using clinical experience?
5. What help could be offered to assist Mrs B in handling her anger?

Case study 2

Mrs C is a 47-year-old lady, married, with two adult children who live locally. She lives in a house which she owns. She has a four-year history of cancer of the bladder, a one-year history of pelvic-bone metastases, and has been known to the palliative care team for nine months.

She had been admitted to hospital for pain control and hypercalcaemia and was fully independent in functional activities on assessment, but the main difficulty identified was extreme discomfort in sitting out of bed due to pain in the pelvic area.

The occupational therapist provided a Roho Quadtro cushion (a pressure-prevention cushion adjustable in four quadrants) and adjusted it with low air level in the rear two quadrants. It was reviewed later the same day and was found not to be providing any relief.

A Burnett cushion, comprising a beanbag-like sac which is shaped to accommodate the user, and whose air could be removed by a pump thus moulding the cushion, was tried. It was hoped that this would provide support but that it could be shaped so that pressure was avoided round the pelvis. Again, this was unsuccessful.

The husband brought in an inflatable ring that Mrs C had been using at home. Mr and Mrs C were made aware of the problems with this – specifically, the tourniquet effect on the buttocks – but as it was only used for short periods and appeared to be the only comfortable solution, it was decided that it would be used.

Mrs C was discharged home but readmitted eight days later for review of pain control. Occupational therapy and physiotherapy reviewed her again regarding mobility and comfort. As she was managing well no further intervention was arranged. Two days prior to being discharge home again, Mrs C developed spinal cord compression at T4 but this was not communicated to the occupational therapist or physiotherapist, nor to the support services going in to assist Mr and Mrs C at home. The nurse in charge on the day of discharge was extremely concerned about their ability to cope at home as Mrs C required one person to help in all transfers.

All the staff and Mrs C's family wanted her to go home as it would be unlikely that she would return home if she did not go on that day. The first the occupational therapist and physiotherapist knew about the situation was when a staff nurse asked for a 'home assessment of some sort' on the morning of the discharge because they were unsure as to whether the home environment would be suitable. This breakdown in communication was extremely unusual for this palliative care team.

The physiotherapist practised safe lifting techniques with the husband on the ward that morning and the occupational therapist discussed the home environment with them to establish any potential hazards. Mr C explained that he had already set up a double bed downstairs with a Spenco mattress (pressure mattress) on his wife's side of the bed. They did not have a commode but the ward loaned them a spare one. One of their neighbours was on the ward visiting Mrs C and she offered to take the commode home while the husband waited for the ambulance to take her home after lunch. In the meantime, the occupational therapist visited the house (with a neighbour present) to ensure that furniture heights and other dimensions were suitable.

The occupational therapist visited the house, all necessary furniture was set up to maintain Mrs C comfortably with district nursing input, and it was decided that a hoist would not be required. This was reported back to the husband and to staff at the hospital, and a follow-up telephone call that evening and the following day ensured that no further intervention was required from the occupational therapist. The occupational therapist also contacted the district nurse to apologize and explain about the circumstances. It was felt important to do this to avoid the community services forming the opinion that such poor organization was commonplace. Once all members of the team were apprised of the situation, they were satisfied that Mrs C's discharge arrangements were safe even though it took place at the last minute.

Discussion points

1. Should the occupational therapist have intervened at such short notice or was this compromising the occupational therapist's professional integrity?
2. Should the occupational therapist have refused on the grounds of unsatisfactory organization on the part of the ward by the 'key workers'? Is the occupational therapist justified in refusing to do this when the client must go home urgently or die in hospital?
3. Whose role was it to pacify staff and allay fears about returning home?
4. Who should have been responsible for telephoning the husband twice after discharge to check that everything was working well?
5. How could such a situation be avoided in future? Which health care professionals should be responsible for co-ordinating discharge plans?

Case study 3

Mr D was a 44-year-old single gentleman. He was unemployed, having previously worked in public relations. Both of his parents had died and he had one sister to whom he was close. He lived in his own ground-floor flat, with level access and no steps indoors.

Mr D had a three-year history of renal cell carcinoma which had been treated with radiotherapy to the right pelvis and, one year later, to the right humerus. On admission, three years after diagnosis, he presented with gross destruction of the right hip joint, widespread disease throughout the pelvis, metastatic disease affecting the right shoulder, and a possible fracture of the right shoulder. His problems on admission were:

- severe pain to the right hip and right shoulder;
- inability to bear weight on the right leg due to instability of the hip joint;
- severely restricted movement at the right shoulder;
- anger;
- suspected depressed mood state.

Chemotherapy was commenced and occupational therapy referral was received three days after admission. Initially, the referral had been:

- to assess for and supply a wheelchair;
- to assess current functional status and Mr D's level of independence;
- to establish whether he needed to return home.

At his initial interview with the occupational therapist, Mr D appeared to be very subdued; he made no eye contact and did not initiate any conversation. When answering questions his replies were monosyllabic, often just 'yes' or 'no' or very short responses. It was very difficult to establish a clear picture of his social situation or of his current functional status as he refused to demonstrate or discuss how he moved from bed to chair and whether he needed any help. When asked directly, he acknowledged that all functional tasks were difficult and accepted that it would be difficult for him to return home without any help. The occupational therapist emphasized the independence rather than the dependence we hoped to achieve and he reluctantly agreed to try an 8L wheelchair (self-propelling with 17" x 17" seat) and 4" Propad (pressure-relieving cushion). He was offered the opportunity to attend the occupational therapy department to look at the range and try out aids to daily living.

Mr D was seen regularly during his hospital admission: he refused any active intervention or to attend the occupational or physiotherapy departments. He preferred to arrange any help himself and remained independent. Nursing staff did report, however, that he required help from one person in washing and dressing himself.

At the weekly multidisciplinary ward meeting, concern was expressed by all members as to how he would cope with his current functional limitations at home but he continued to refuse any referrals to the community services.

The nursing staff who worked most closely with Mr D felt he should be made to attend the occupational therapy department and told him he must attend. He refused. They also informed him that social worker and community liaison would see him but only told him five minutes before they arrived and he refused to see them. He agreed to see the social worker the following day and community support was suggested and arranged with his agreement.

The occupational therapist referred him to his local wheelchair clinic for a permanent wheelchair and a pressure-relieving cushion; this referral was accepted but the wheelchair clinic had also received a referral from Mr D's general practitioner requesting provision of an electric wheelchair. As it was unlikely that Mr D was aware of the GP's referral, the occupational therapist asked the wheelchair clinic to put it on hold until she had spoken to him. She asked the nursing staff if Mr D had mentioned an electric wheelchair to them and they said no but they thought it was a very good idea. When asked why it would be a good idea, they were not sure. Mr D was less impressed by the idea of an electric wheelchair and declined it firmly. The wheelchair clinic and GP were informed of this.

Mr D was discharged home, self-medicating and independent in his wheelchair. He accepted referrals to the district nurses and home care. Although his pain control was much improved:

- his right leg remained unable to bear weight as the right hip was crumbling;
- he remained wheelchair dependent;
- he remained fatigued;
- he remained unable to move his right shoulder – he was therefore functionally impaired as his right hand was dominant;
- he required one person's help in order to wash and dress;
- he needed a hoist to transfer him in and out of the bath;
- he remained dependent on help from one person to manage domestic tasks.

Discussion points

1. Should the occupational therapist and team have insisted that Mr D attend the department for full assessment?

2. Should the occupational therapist have insisted that a referral be made to the community occupational therapy service?
3. Outline a treatment programme to facilitate Mr D's optimal independence if he had chosen to be co-operative.
4. What support could be given to the multidisciplinary team to avoid different health care professionals being in conflict with each other over the management of this case?
5. What issues does this case raise concerning the client's autonomy?

Case study 4

Miss H was a 45-year-old single lady. She had her own basement flat, which was accessible via six outside steps and was level indoors. She had no family living locally but she had a very supportive network of friends. Her work colleagues at the local council offices had been very helpful.

Miss H was diagnosed with right breast cancer four years ago, when she had a partial mastectomy, axillary clearance, adjuvant chemotherapy, radiotherapy and then placed on a five-year trial of Tamoxifen (an anti-breast-cancer drug). One year after the initial diagnosis, a further right-breast mass was discovered and surgically removed. Supraclavicular fossa nodes were treated with chemotherapy. Two years after that episode, the disease recurred in the breast, supraclavicular fossa nodes, axillary nodes and the cervical spine, and bony metastases were observed in the right femur.

She was admitted under the palliative care team for radiotherapy to the spine. Occupational therapy assessment identified no functional difficulties despite the fact that she presented with mild right-upper-limb lymphoedema and was right-hand dominant. After seven days in hospital for radiotherapy Miss H was discharged home with no services set up as she had refused all help.

The occupational therapist felt bath transfers would be steadier and safer using a bath or shower board but Miss H viewed this in a negative light as it highlighted her impairment. The occupational therapist offered her assistance if she felt it would be useful but agreed with the client that it was her choice not to accept it at this stage.

Miss H was readmitted two days later with poorly controlled pain and an unstable neck at C3/4. A hard collar was immediately fitted. Miss H was reluctant to wear this, although she had been advised of the potential risk of paralysis. She had intended to go on holiday with two friends six days after the most recent hospital admission and failed to accept that this was not feasible due to the need for pain control.

In order to plan for discharge home once symptoms were adequately controlled, the occupational therapist carried out a full functional assessment. The main difficulties were identified as lifting the kettle, transferring food in and out of the oven, and bath transfers. Alternative techniques for filling and using the kettle and oven were acceptable – for example, boiling a mug of water and preparing meals in the microwave. Although Miss H accepted a referral to the local social services for bathing equipment, she would not accept the same equipment in hospital.

The ward staff found her constant refusal of help, which they perceived as essential, to be frustrating. Her negative view of rehabilitation as reinforcing disability resulted in her acquiring the 'unpopular and difficult patient' label. The ward staff responded by constantly asking the occupational therapist and physiotherapist 'Can't you offer anything to rehabilitate her?' She would shower alone on the ward, lock the door, refuse staff access and contradict herself by agreeing that not wearing the collar could cause paralysis but still choosing not to do so.

Two days prior to the holiday, Miss H agreed it would be unfair on her friends if she were to go. Discharge home was not appropriate due to ongoing treatment and the plan was to move her to an appropriate unit nearer home so that her friends could visit.

Her altered body image involved:

- being unable to wear contact lenses due to decreased range of movement and lymphoedema of the upper limb;
- being unable to undertake tasks she would have managed previously;
- hair loss due to radiotherapy;
- decreased mobility.

Instead of focusing her care on key workers, Miss H was referred to more professionals. Miss H had visited a local hospice one weekend unknown to either the hospital or the hospice staff and reported that she did not like it. She had not discussed her care or the support services available there so this was investigated at a full case conference.

She did transfer to the hospice after the meeting at which future plans and areas of specific help were identified.

Discussion points

1. Should the issues of patient autonomy and professional assessment result in conflict and how can they be resolved?
2. Could the occupational therapist have used an alternative approach to introduce equipment to Miss H, emphasizing its positive aspects?
3. How could the multidisciplinary team address and plan for future needs when Miss H was unrealistic and inaccurate about her own abilities?
4. Discuss how to approach her altered body image.

Case study 5

Mr J was a 31-year-old man, who was unemployed, divorced for three years, and living in a shared house with three other single men. He had had a lump on his left hand for 20 years and nothing was ever done about it. Four years ago it was excised and a biopsy showed it was benign. One year ago it recurred and was excised but was found to have malignant cells.

Referral was received from physiotherapy the day before surgery, the plan being for removal of little and ring fingers, portion of arm on the ulnar border to the wrist (involving metacarpals, carpal bones and ulnar head) followed by two weeks radiotherapy. He was seen prior to surgery to discuss his daily routine, his main functional difficulties prior to admission, and his main concerns.

Mr J was chiefly concerned regarding driving and future limb fitting/prosthesis.

Contact was maintained post-surgery as he was gradually encouraged to do as much as possible given that he had drains and bandages *in situ*. His walking was unaffected and all transfers including moving in and out of the bath were independent, although drying himself was reported to be time-consuming.

He was seen in the occupational therapy department where one-handed equipment was demonstrated, although it was emphasized that he should regain more use of the left hand as treatment progressed and equipment would, hopefully, not be required later on. With regard to his cooking, prior to admission he either obtained a takeaway or walked to the local cafe. He had use of a microwave and felt opening cans would be difficult.

He took his laundry to a local laundrette for a service wash and did not do a significant amount of shopping.

He was on invalidity benefit and the social worker ensured that all benefits were applied for.

Once the drains and bandaging were removed, the only equipment he needed was one-handed cutlery as the left hand was still too sore to grip. Mr J appeared to show little interest in his discharge home. He was not satisfied with his domestic arrangements and realized that he was the only one who could improve them but felt little motivation to do so. The social worker requested the occupational therapist prepare a functional report for benefits.

Mr J had claimed he needed the help of one person in all activities in the part he had filled in. The occupational therapist provided an objective report identifying that no assistance was required and the social worker was unhappy that this would prevent him from receiving the full amount of benefits. The occupational therapist, however, was not prepared to change the report to support his claims.

He was discharged to a specialist orthopaedic hospital nearer his home where he continued to see the hand therapist and apparently began to see a counsellor.

Discussion points

1. Identify the functional implications of the loss of the ulnar aspect of the non-dominant hand.
2. Describe the occupational therapy intervention programme in the short and long term to assist in his rehabilitation.
3. What are the ethical and moral considerations of the occupational therapist being asked to change the functional report in order to increase the chances of Mr J receiving maximum benefits?

Case study 6

Mrs W was a 67-year-old married woman, living with her husband in their own house. Their five adult children lived nearby and they were involved with a local church, the congregation being very supportive and helpful. She presented with a four-year history of visual loss, and was diagnosed in February 1996 as having a pituitary adenoma. Surgery was performed to debulk the tumour and decompress the optic nerve. One of the risks of this surgery was possible damage to the optic nerve. Sadly this did take place and permanent blindness occurred. Mrs W was to remain in hospital for six weeks' radiotherapy.

Occupational therapy assessment concentrated on functional independence in the ward setting commencing with personal care, eating and orientation towards managing in her own room. She initially appeared reluctant to use a cane or stick and was encouraged to physically explore her room, touching the furniture, and so forth. She and her family were understandably grieving for her loss of sight and the staff all helped them in coming to terms with this. This was felt to be a healthy grieving process and specific counselling was not required.

There was the added social complication of the family having lodgers – three adult gentlemen with learning disabilities who had been discharged into the community from an institution. Mrs W felt guilty at the prospect of the lodgers needing to find alternative accommodation. The social worker became involved in order to help rehouse them. Referral was also made to the rehabilitation officer for visual impairment and a case conference was organized inviting the social worker, the rehabilitation officer and the general practitioner into the hospital to discuss discharge planning.

All the staff involved were made aware of the importance of maintaining Mrs W's environment as constant as possible, particularly the domestics, who were requested not to move the furniture.

The occupational therapist carried out a home assessment with Mr and Mrs W present, and successfully guided her round the house and practised a few steps orientating herself round the lounge. She proceeded to have weekend leave which was very successful and this helped to improve her self-esteem and her confidence. However, she did express concern regarding how her husband was coping emotionally and she was also worried about having too many visitors at weekends, even though they were well meaning. She was advised to give friends clear guidelines on the number of visitors who could come and encourage them to make a rota, which proved to be useful.

Mrs W was discharged home with follow-up and continuing care from the rehabilitation officer for the visually impaired.

Discussion points

1. Outline the occupational therapy treatment programme for this lady suggesting any equipment and techniques to deal with this traumatic disability.
2. How could the team assist the husband to cope emotionally? To whom might he be referred for help?
3. What will the future and ongoing needs be for this lady and her family?

* * * * * *

Appendix 15 Screening Tool for Referral to Occupational Therapist

The 'screening tool' provided below was devised by the UK Occupational Therapist Specialist Section HOPE (HIV/AIDS, Oncology, Palliative Care and Education) and can assist carers in deciding when referral to an occupational therapist might be needed. It should not, however, be used to assess the needs of clients – the assessment of function and dysfunction is the task of the occupational therapist. Often a colleague refers someone for help – for example, with bathing aids – only for the occupational therapist to discover a range of previously unidentified functional difficulties.

SCREENING TOOL re FUNCTION

This is NOT an assessment, but a means of identifying the need for referral on to Occupational Therapy.
If any areas identified in the last column, please refer to Occupational therapy . If no direct access to this service, contact local hospital O.T.
Department or Social Services O.T. Department.

DO YOU HAVE ANY PROBLEMS WITH ACTIVITIES SUCH AS: –	NO	YES, BUT HAVE OVERCOME DIFFICULTY	YES, REQUIRE ADVICE RE. ALTERNATIVE TECHNIQUE/EQUIPMENT
WASHING including cleaning teeth, wringing out flannel DRESSING including putting on underwear BATHING/USING WC. including washing hair			
KITCHEN ACTIVITIES including peeling potatoes, hanging out washing WRITING/USING KEYBOARD EATING including managing cutlery			
WALKING USING STAIRS TRANSFERS e.g. in/out of bed or bath			
WORKING i.e. job, profession LEISURE including holding cards, gardening DRIVING/TRANSPORT including turning key, managing pedals			
ANY OTHER AREAS OF LIFE:			
DO YOU REQUIRE ADVICE/HELP WITH ANY PROBLEMS?			

Appendix 16
Preventing Cancer

In October 1995, the European Commission's campaign against cancer issued the following guidelines for cancer prevention:

1. Do not smoke. Smokers, stop as quickly as possible and do not smoke in the presence of others. If you do not smoke, do not try it.
2. If you drink alcohol, whether beer, wine or spirits, moderate your consumption.
3. Increase your daily intake of vegetables and fresh fruit. Eat cereals with a high fibre content frequently.
4. Avoid becoming overweight, increase physical activity and limit intake of fatty foods.
5. Avoid excessive exposure to the sun and avoid sunburn especially in children.
6. Apply strictly regulations aimed at preventing any exposure to known cancer-causing substances. Follow all health and safety instructions on substances which may cause cancer. More cancers may be cured if detected early.
7. See your doctor if you notice a lump, a sore which does not heal (including one in the mouth), a mole which changes in shape, size or colour, or any abnormal bleeding.
8. See your doctor if you have persistent problems, such as a persistent cough, persistent hoarseness, a change in bowel or urinary habits or an unexplained weight loss.
9. If you are a woman, have a cervical smear regularly and participate in an organized screening programme for cervical cancer.
10. Check your breasts regularly. Participate in organized mammographic screening programmes if you are over 50.

* * * * * *

Glossary

Aesthesia is perception, feeling or sensation.

Anaplasia is a characteristic of tumour tissue where there is loss of differentiation of cells and their orientation to one another.

Adenocarcinomas arise from the cells of tissues in which glandular structures are common features – for example, the thyroid gland, stomach or pancreas.

Cachexia is a marked state of malnutrition and general ill health.

Carpal tunnel syndrome presents as a complex of symptoms resulting from compression of the median nerve in the carpal tunnel, with pain and burning or tingling parasthesias in the fingers and hand up to the elbow.

Cognition involves the ability of the mind to perceive, think and remember.

CVA is a cerebrovascular accident or stroke.

Demyelination is loss, removal or destruction of the myelin sheath surrounding nerves.

Denervation is resection or removal of the nerves to an organ or part.

Dyspnoea is difficult or laboured breathing.

Dyspraxia is partial loss of ability to perform co-ordinated acts. For example, dressing dyspraxia might involve difficulty in recognizing body parts and clothing.

Dysfunction is difficulty in normal action, disturbance or impairment to functioning of an organ.

Dysphagia is difficulty in swallowing.

Dysphasia refers to impairment in speech due to lack of co-ordination and an inability to find words.

Ergonomics is the science relating individuals to their environment in order to achieve the most efficient use of energy or resources.

Ewing's sarcoma is a highly malignant metastatic tumour of the primitive small round cells of the bone, usually occurring in the diaphyses of long bones, ribs and flat bones of children or adolescents.

Hemiparesis is partial paralysis or weakness affecting one side of the body.

Hemiplegia is paralysis of one side of the body.

Hyperaesthesia is disturbance in sensation resulting in increased sensitivity, particularly a painful sensation from a normally painless touch stimulus.

Hypercalcaemia is excess of calcium in the blood resulting in fatigue, muscle weakness, depression, anorexia, nausea and constipation.

Leiomyosarcomas are primary tumours in smooth muscle – in the uterus for example.

Leukaemia is a progressive malignant disease of the blood-forming organs, characterized by distorted proliferation and development of leukocytes and their precursors in the blood and bone marrow.

Lymphoma is abnormal growth of lymphoid tissue or cancer developing from cells in the lymphatic system.

Lymphoedema is the accumulation of lymph fluid in the tissues resulting in swelling caused by obstruction of the lymphatic vessels.

Melanoma is a tumour arising from the melanocytic system of the skin and other organs. When used alone the term often refers to malignant melanoma.

Myeloma is a tumour composed of cells of the type normally found in the bone marrow.

Neuropathy is a functional disturbance or pathological change in the peripheral nervous system.

Neutropenia refers to a decrease in the number of neutrophilic leukocytes in the blood resulting in susceptibility to infections.

Oedema is the excessive accumulation of fluid in body tissues.

Oncology is the study and practice of treating tumours.

Paraesthesia is abnormal touch sensation, for example burning or pricking, often in the absence of external stimuli.

Pathological fractures occur when bone is weakened by disease, such as a tumour.

Peripheral neuropathy (also known as multiple neuropathy or polyneuropathy) is the neuropathy of several peripheral nerves simultaneously.

Pneumonitis is inflammation of the lungs.

Postherpetic neuralgia is persistent burning pain and hyperaesthesia along the distribution of a cutaneous nerve following an attack of herpes zoster.

Proprioception is the information provided by specialized sensory nerve endings in the joints monitoring muscle and tendon activity indicating joint positions in space.

Pruritis is itching. So uraemic pruritis, for example, is generalized itching associated with chronic renal failure and not related to other internal or skin disease,

Rhabdomyosarcomas are malignant tumours of 'striped' muscle such as that of the thigh or arm. They are most commonly seen in adolescents.

Sarcomas are primary cancer growths in soft tissue and occasionally bone.

Squamous cell carcinoma is a malignant tumour originating from an organ with a surface or lining epithelium of cells – for example, the bronchus or oesophagus.

* * * * * *

Index